Raising Three Daughters While
Dancing Around Death and Divorce

PLANETS, TRANSPLANTS, AND AUTOCORRECT

DOUGLAS SWINFORD

This work depicts actual events in the life of the author as truthfully as recollection permits. While all persons within are actual individuals, some names and identifying characteristics have been changed to respect their privacy.

ISBN: 979-8-9853914-4-2

Published by Rorie Lynne

Contact the author at dmichael13@comcast.net

First edition 2023

In Loving Memory of my parents

Barb (1933-2022) and Dale (1930-2014) Swinford

CONTENTS

PREFACE

I first met Douglas Swinford early in my career at Carle Clinic, Urbana, Illinois, as a Gastrointestinal Consultant in August 1984, when he was 24 years old. He was referred to me because of an unknown liver disease and anemia, which he had been suffering from for the past year.

At that time, he was married and had an eight-month-old daughter, eventually followed by a second daughter in 1985 and a third daughter in 1989.

I shortly confirmed the diagnosis of Primary Sclerosing Cholangitis (PSC) associated with ulcerative colitis and shared a thorough and honest discussion with Douglas and his wife. I emphasized to them that his condition was chronic, incurable, and would probably require a liver transplant in the future. I stressed the financial medical burden, the need for frequent medical testing and medications, and the psychological impact on Doug and his wife. Despite this, Douglas continued working at Illinois Power Company, now Ameren, and deferred disability. Douglas resolved that he would not let these factors deter his responsibility of mentoring his young daughters.

As predicted, he dealt with progressive liver problems, life-threatening internal bleeding episodes, and debilitating fevers and finally underwent the first of three liver transplants in 1991. Shortly after the first transplant, he and his wife divorced, and Douglas obtained custody of his three young daughters, which he raised to adulthood with the help of their mother and his family.

His first transplant lasted 13 years, but due to a recurrence of PSC, he required a second transplant in 2004. Complications were a gradual recurrence of PSC, a plasma cell tumor in the colon, and eventually liver failure. Long-term use of immune suppression medication compromised the kidneys to the point that he required dialysis in early 2020. Multiple organ failure led to a rare third liver transplant in July 2020, followed shortly by a kidney transplant. Throughout this 29-year medical ordeal, Douglas continued to work full time and to function as a single parent raising three daughters through adolescence to successful adulthood.

Douglas continuously impresses me with his deep religious faith, his love for life, and his love for and from his family.

He reminds me of the Biblical story of Job. He accepted the multiple episodes of disastrous financial and medical complications; he continues to overcome what comes his way with a calm but intelligent acceptance rooted in a deep resolve not to let anything prevent or destroy his love of life or his conviction that his purpose is to help others. I am grateful for the time I have spent with Douglas. I suggest that others with chronic, incurable diseases will benefit from reading his memoir, particularly learning of the empowerment of his love and life-long humanitarian motives. For years, I have displayed a plaque in my office with a quotation of the famous 15th-century physician Ambrose Pare, c.1510-1590:

"I treated him, God cured him."

I am not sure what the future will hold for Douglas Swinford. However, based on his history, when all is said and done, I am sure he will have had a beautiful and bountiful life, setting an example for all to follow. His journey illustrates to others that life is not influenced by the tragedies that occur but rather by how one reacts to them.

Signed
Dr. Eugene Greenberg
Institute of Digestive Health,
Carle Clinic Urbana, Illinois

Chapter 1

Dying to Live, July 14, 2020

I dismissed sleep because if I was going to die, I wanted to at least be awake for it. No one wants to miss a wedding, the birth of a child, or any major life event. Death is the big one because it is the last act.

I had come this close to getting help. I didn't want a *coup fourré* of death sneaking in. Tomorrow was going to be consequential.

I was at Barnes-Jewish Hospital in St. Louis, Missouri, to receive a liver and kidney transplant. The liver was the real culprit. I knew that dialysis could step in for failed kidneys. Dialysis felt like being stranded on an island with only one person to date. There was no attraction at all. But if you didn't date her, she would kill you. I entered this relationship with Di on January 17, 2020. The miserable swelling of ankles and fatigue persisted. But I lived to fight another day.

Liver disease delivers some of the worst experiences humans can endure. Eyes and skin turning yellow, itching, and an inability to sleep are just tune-ups. Deeper in the pool, liver disease leads to life-threatening internal bleeding, dramatically presented from the mouth or the digestive system.

In the lead-up to the transplant, I was hospitalized for such a bleed on May 29, 2020. My liver became unable to help stop the internal bleeding. At the same time, it started failing to remove toxins, particularly ammonia, from the bloodstream. As the toxins rose that day, Hepatic Encephalopathy crept up to a crescendo. This date was also my eighth wedding anniversary with my wife, Lynne. No romantic dinners to recall our scenic wedding just off the coast of the Pacific at Waimanalo, on the Hawaiian island of Oahu. Instead, I woke up that day at Barnes-Jewish Hospital. I felt a little confused and had no idea how long I had been there. The nurse said, "Mr. Douglas, your daughter Jessica called and said not to forget that today is a special day and that she and Lynne are staying at the nearby Parkway Hotel. She will try to call you today, so don't forget to wish her Happy Anniversary." The nurse followed with, "We are sorry, Mr. Douglas, that she can't come and see you, but you are aware of the restrictions due to the COVID pandemic."

I was dismayed but not surprised that I couldn't see my wife, but I had started getting accustomed to the isolation. The doctor making rounds that morning asked me, "Mr. Swinford, do you know what day of the week it is? Do you know where you are? How long do you think you have been here?"

"I am in Barnes Hospital." My other guesses were way off,

and it upset me that I didn't know the simplest of things.

"We are going to increase your lactulose to help clear your mind." I disliked this overly sweet medicine that I was to drink. It accelerated my digestive system, helped the body rid itself of poisons, and kept down the toxic effects on my brain.

By the time the medicine arrived, a paranoia formed in my mind that my family was in jeopardy. I saw threatening symbols on the television. In my thinking, to protect my family, I needed to refuse the medicine. Usually, I've always been a tranquil and compliant patient, but in my state of mind, I started seeing the nurses as adversaries.

"Mr. Swinford, you *have* to drink this!"

"You are going to get more confused, and can go into a coma!"

As the day wore on, hospital staff made various efforts to deliver the medicine. Locked in my alternate world, I had the adrenaline and strength to resist, and in doing so, I thought it would help the kids survive. All imaginary, but like a computer with a virus, my ability to reason had short-circuited. I also found it very hard to stand or walk, like being very drunk and having poor motor skills.

Having exhausted all reasonable options, two nurses came in and discussed how to proceed. "Mr. Swinford, you have refused all day to take your medicine. We understand your daughter is a nurse practitioner, and we are going to call her and discuss how critical it is to get you to comply."

In short order, they used my phone and reached her at a nearby restaurant where she and my wife were dining. They had her on Facetime. "Dad, please do as the nurses are asking!" She saw a blank stare looking back at her and asked to speak with the nurses. "I know how serious this is. Would you please consider letting my step-mom Lynne in to see if she can help get him to obey?"

The nurses then asked me if I would take my medicine if my wife came in.

"Yes." But I had no plan of doing so. While hepatic encephalopathy clouded my thinking, it elevated my cunning and manipulation skills. I would say anything I needed to say. I intended to let her in on the secret mission to help save our family; thus, she could help remedy the crisis in my imagination. Imagine my upset with my wife when she came in and didn't understand. She *also* insisted on me taking the medicine. The last thing I remembered was ending up in a quasi-wrestling match with the nurses trying to get a syringe full of lactulose between my clenched teeth.

My wife stayed calm, but her heartbreak was evident. Anniversaries are supposed to be happy occasions. Liver disease was playing the trump card, and I was entering dangerous territory as I mercifully lost consciousness. I woke the next morning wearing "boxing gloves," officially called "safety mittens," meant for unruly patients. On the positive side, I had forgotten the rest of the events from the night before, and with a clear mind, I was fully cooperative.

After that dreadful episode and less severe bouts of mental confusion over the next four weeks, we were nearing a crossroads. The looming question was, what further, if anything, could be done for me? Thus, came the conversation with someone I will refer to as "Coach." Sitting alone in my hospital room at Barnes, after a two-month slide towards going on to my "reward," as they called it in the old days, I was just getting acquainted with an episode of *Forensic Files*. I'd just undergone a rigorous day of testing to see if I would qualify for a liver and kidney transplant. Coach entered the room, closed the door, introduced herself, and announced she had important matters to discuss.

Oh no, I thought to myself, *is she going to tell me that I am too sick for a transplant?*

At this point, no one had told me how my tests were going and if I would qualify for a transplant. Two years prior, I did the workup at Barnes for a kidney transplant. I received a letter that said something like: "Mr. Swinford, we regret to inform you that you do not qualify for a kidney transplant. You have marked liver disease of a severity that transplant is not an option for you."

Okay, I understood that then, and now we were asking for both organs. Surely, Coach wouldn't tell me that news when I was by myself. But in the age of COVID-19, they rarely let family in. That news would mean the struggle was over. No more tests. All of the efforts would be for my comfort. Within days or maybe a few weeks, I would slip into a coma, and it would be over. As I held my breath, she said, "Mr. Swinford, I am an anesthesiologist with the transplant team, and our job is to keep you asleep and allow the work to be done."

I breathed a little easier as this sounded more like I would receive help.

"Mr. Swinford, this is going to be the hardest thing you have ever done. You will have to give everything you have to survive this!"

I nodded my head that I understood.

She went on, "I see that you have had two previous liver transplants in 1991 and 2004. This is different. The surgeons have indicated that it is very rare to get a third liver. Your scar tissue, adhesions, and kidney failure make this more difficult." She halted briefly, then continued, "You will feel like you have been run over by a truck. There will be adversity. If you can't fight through the inevitable setbacks, you won't make it." She looked at me with an intensity born out of experience. To make her point, she paused again as if to let the words soak in.

Was I being evaluated to see if I had the fortitude to do this? Was this a pep talk? I returned her look with acceptance and sincerity. I assured her I understood what was being asked of me. She seemed satisfied that she had delivered her message and was on her way.

If I were honest with myself, I had doubts about whether I

could pull through during this sick, sicker, and as-sick-as-you-can-be-and-still-be-alive period of the last few months. I was experiencing strange activity. When I closed my eyes, I saw these brilliant lights with colors so bright as to seem other-worldly. Other times, I saw the clear night sky with all the stars, Milky Way, and planets as if I was in a planetarium or some very dark corner of the Earth. In my potpourri of visions, hallucinations, or whatever I was experiencing… also came the numbers. Digital numbers like you would see on a car odometer, but spinning like on a slot machine, going around and around and stopping. When I saw the numbers, they were on the right. A baseball field was on the left. Perhaps I was seeing the old-time scoreboards at ballparks that cropped in the corner of my mind, as if in a dream where odd connections appear. But this was no dream.

Earlier in the day, before Coach came, I had asked a doctor about the lights I kept seeing. "Douglas, I think it is related to the retina surgery in your left eye."

I didn't bother to tell him the colorful visions had been visible in both eyes for months prior to the surgery. And what did I really expect him to say? "Yes, Douglas, patients tell me about the bright lights they see all the time right before they cash in their chips!"

No, he wasn't going to tell me that, even if it was true. Now, if it was Coach, she would give it to me straight. "Sir, we often find that patients see lights right before they perish, so stop closing your eyes!"

I might see her again at surgery time. I liked her. Give it to me straight, Coach. I know I'm in a hell of a shape.

I felt like a boxer with a big fight the next day. I knew I was going to get my ass kicked. However, I knew firsthand that I would have to suck it up for a few days and use all the hydrocodone and Dilaudid they offered; before long, I would start to feel better. If all went well, I would experience the absolutely amazing transformation that successful organ transplants could deliver.

Even with imperfections, transplants extend the life and often a lot of quality of life if the patient takes care of their end of the job, which is a substantial commitment in itself.

I just wanted to get rebuilt with donated organs, get out of the hospital, and be in the comfort of my home. I hoped to get back to a normal life. Coach actually helped me believe that I had a chance to do just that. She wouldn't waste her time if she wasn't in the know that it was likely that I would be on the list. Little did she or I know, but the listing and the "call" would both come within 14 days of our meeting.

The nurse entered my hospital room and exclaimed, "Mr. Douglas, you really need to get some sleep!" Her tone hinted at a mild scolding, not a serious reprimand. She continued, "This will be a long surgery. We want to send you down to the OR having had some rest!" All the nurses treated me extra nicely, knowing what a challenging situation I faced and how the pending operation only marked the beginning of a long climb, assuming I could make it through.

A sense of relief came with knowing that this ordeal was coming to a conclusion. We would know if this situation was salvageable within the next few days and weeks. I knew it couldn't keep going like this with cycles of encephalopathy kidnapping me for days at a time. When I emerged from the fog, I would get so low, mainly from feeling terrible. On the rare occasion she was allowed to see me, my wife Lynne would try to sing Hawaiian songs that I loved from her background in the Philippines and Hawaii to encourage me. She also implored me to keep going. "Honey, you have to do this for the kids and grandkids!"

Even in my low points, I held onto an unspoken obligation to keep trying. What if I didn't want to keep going? What if I had my fill of this suffering? Didn't I have the right to get released from this predicament? Did anyone have any idea of the misery involved to keep living with organ failure? All of the common pleasures of life were gone. I rarely got to eat regular food. Instead, it was some form of gruel or tasteless broth. Even a good drink of water or ice chips might be off-limits at times, and the only drink I could get was a pasty liquid so they could take pictures of my inner workings. This wasn't living; this was merely existing.

I believed God was the ultimate arbitrator, yet even in prayer, I didn't have as good of a case as I did in my younger years. In 1991, my daughters were only seven years, five years, and 20 months old. I just had to survive to be a part of their support and raising. For my transplant in 2004, there still existed a lot of work to do in my career and raising my children. But then, my health had already ended my work career. The girls had all graduated college already. I had walked them down the aisle at their weddings. The grandchildren were a wonderful part of life. Despite battling disease and fighting off early calls from the grim reaper, I had been able to have a full life. For this transplant in 2020, I felt more accepting of what might come…

But then I would get this feeling inside—imagine the pressure before a geyser bursts. When I thought about the assassination attempts by this damned disease, fury welled up inside of me, and chills ran up my spine. I felt so stubbornly defiant to have my life end.

It could be called survival instinct. My personal belief is that the life breathed into me by God is an event not easily extinguished. While seriously ill, I was in the right time and the right place. Was it possible that I was capable of withstanding more than I thought I could? Even after a two-month slide spent in and out of the hospital and many days in the ICU, where all dignity was surrendered? Yes, even as the separation from my loved ones prevailed.

So I stayed vigilant through the night. Transport came to take me down to pre-op at 4:30 a.m., and my thoughts went back to the start of it all, many years ago on a nice summer day.

CHAPTER 2

CHALLENGES OF A YOUNG FAMILY

What could cause the need for four organ replacements in 29 years? I was just a regular guy going to a regular job on September 1, 1983. I was married with a baby on the way, and we had just purchased our first home. Just getting a good start in life.

I worked for Illinois Power Co.—the local utility company. We were digging to run a gas service line to a building on the University of Illinois campus. The hum of the traffic and laughter of the students making their way to class on the tree-lined campus served as background music for our job.

My crew leader, Phil Cochrane, said, "Hey, Dougie, cut off the pipe where I marked it."

"Okay. I'll grab the wire cutters to cut the locate wire, too." I felt a sharp pain in my abdomen. I tried to shake it off and took a couple of Tylenol. To be on Phil's crew was the best assignment I could hope to get. He was tall and carried an air of confidence. His sense of humor and storytelling skills were unmatched. Most importantly, he actually took the time to train us young guys and let us operate the equipment. The old timers thought the only tools an apprentice needed was a spade, a shovel, and a putty knife. I had just concluded to myself, *There is no way I'm leaving this job*.

Phil picked up on my distress. "What's the problem, Dougie? You look a little peaked."

"Phil, my belly hurts so bad. I can't shake it."

Within an hour, I sat in the small waiting room of our family physician Dr. Martin Koeck's office. He had known and taken care of me since I was born. The room smelled of cleaner, but I always tried to identify the other smell that seemed typical in medical settings. Like a room full of vitamins lay just out of sight. Whatever it was, it had never changed, nor had the stack of magazines, such as *Reader's Digest* and *Highlights* for kids near their little play area. As a kid, I knew a dum-dum lollipop was mine if I was brave while getting a shot. It was a comfortable place.

Once in the exam room, Dr. Koeck assessed me quickly and stated, "Doug, I'm going to send you to the hospital. Your symptoms of firmness in the area of your liver and the hint of jaundice in your eyes need to be investigated." He seemed almost a bit shaken by what he saw.

By that evening and after numerous tests, a doctor came in to consult with me. "Sir, your condition is quite concerning. You have hepatitis or inflammation of the liver, and we are trying to find the cause. It could be any number of viral diseases or even cancer."

This news came as quite a shock. I was only 23 years old. But it was no different from what happened to people every day when a middle-aged man listened as his doctor explained, "Dear Mr. Jones, I'm sorry to inform you, but you have a brain tumor." Or "Dear Ms. Smith, I'm sorry to tell you that you have breast cancer." Yes, it happened every day; it was just not supposed to happen to *me*.

But it was happening to me. That night, in the hospital, after my wife had gone home and the lights were low, I dragged my IV pole to the restroom and fell to my knees. "Dear God, am I going to die soon?" I asked myself, *did I do something to deserve this?* I knew I was flawed and had made my share of foolish mistakes in the beer-drinking, hell-raising, girl-chasing selfishness of my youth, but to be so sick so soon? I felt like a baseball player who made a couple of errors in the first two innings of the game and was taken out before I could redeem myself. Badly shaken, the infallibility of youth vanished in an instant. It wasn't a "St. Peter on the road to Damascus" moment, but the awareness of a spiritual realm and something bigger beyond what I had known became very present. I had exited the physical into the spiritual, even though I was not in a great position to do so. I knew only what I had learned in my very light church efforts to this point. The late pastor and author Dr. Norman Vincent Peale described the spiritual realm like the blades of a fan. You cannot really see the blades when the fan is running, but when you turn it off, it comes into clear view. That invisible realm was now visible to me. I had to make that adjustment quickly. Fortunately, they didn't come up with any diagnosis that would send me into this unknown anytime soon. I was released a couple of days later and told to follow up with my specialist.

The incident passed, and I was able to return to work. The health scare didn't take long to get put on the back burner. We moved in the winter of 1983, and Debby, my first wife, was having a difficult pregnancy. By Christmas Eve morning, I woke to my wife holding her lower back. "I think these contractions are the real thing!"

Oh no, I thought. The wind had howled ferociously all night long and blew the snow into dune-like drifts all around our home. Record low wind chill moved in after the snow. The news advised against travel due to road closures. Always dependable Dr. Koeck, who had been part of my recent situation, was snowbound in town. We sat in our modest two-bedroom home with a nursery all set up and ready. We had planned for everything except this. We were advised to get in close proximity to the hospital and report contractions. I didn't really know what to do, but I called my parents, who lived nearby, and my mom made some calls. Fortunately, in small-town life word travels fast, and a local businessman named Mike Pierce offered to take us to the hospital in his four-wheel-drive truck. For insurance, he put a snowmobile in the back if the roads weren't passable.

He definitely utilized the four-wheel-drive capabilities of his truck as he maneuvered around snow drifts and stuck cars, but thankfully, the snowmobile went unneeded. We arrived safely at my brother Gary and his wife Debbie's home near the hospital.

We later skidded to the hospital, and at 4:22 a.m. on Christmas Day, our first daughter, Ashley, was born. As soon as I saw her and held her, I was changed. Her birth began to crack the shell of my selfishness to help me be a better person. The introduction of a child became an ally against this disease which my doctors were still trying to figure out.

We had the baby, and I was working. At times I seemed to feel the symptoms and more fatigue. Other times, everything seemed normal. It was easy to forget, but at times, fevers from no other apparent cause reminded me that an unknown issue lurked in the background. I met with my liver specialist in late August 1984, and he confessed, "Doug, I just can't figure out what your problem is. I'd like to refer you to Dr. Eugene Greenberg at Carle Clinic. He has more experience with this sort of matter than I do." He was from India, with a delightful accent to break this news to me. I appreciated him being so forthcoming. He had been so kind all along.

A couple of weeks later, I sat nervously in Dr. Eugene Greenberg's exam room. I had never met the man. After a slight knock, he entered, sharply dressed in slacks and a stylish shirt. "What are you here for?" he said. He studied the lab work and notes in my chart carefully.

I started, "Dr. Greenberg, we have been at this for almost a year. I have been examined by multiple specialists. My labs are up and down. No one seems to know what is going on."

He had me lie down and, while prodding me, asked the standard questions like, "Does this hurt here?" The dialogue felt pointed, and I felt like someone on the stand during a court case. He paused and looked at me long as if he was trying to "read" me. His reputation, by all accounts, suggested that he was an extraordinary physician. With that, he was probably very wise regarding drug and alcohol abuse because either could cause my symptoms. Looking directly in my eyes, he said in a serious, don't give me any B.S. tone, "Do you drink alcohol?"

"No, sir."

He continued, "When was the last time you had any alcohol?"

I was sure he had heard all manner of lies, excuses, and dodges. "Dr. Greenberg, I can assure you that I have not been drinking. My drinking career was limited, mostly when running around with buddies before getting married at 21. After getting sick at 23, and told that I had a problem with my liver, I quit completely." I fibbed a little, leaving out that I had a sip of wine on special occasions and a shot of tequila on my birthday. Not enough to affect anything. I was prepared to stop those, too, if it was detrimental in any way.

He mulled over my responses and returned his gaze to my chart. Satisfied with my answers, he thought and studied for what felt like an eternity as I sat there in silence. He finally said, "I think we are dealing with primary sclerosing cholangitis. I will set up further testing and an exploratory biopsy to clarify."

I was surprised and taken aback but had questions, too. "Dr. Greenberg, can you tell me what causes this disease and what the treatment is?"

"It is a serious disease. We believe it to be an autoimmune disorder, and the disease causes your bile ducts to be damaged. There are no known causal factors. The prognosis is poor, but this can develop slowly. We only came into treatment in recent years with a liver transplant. It is becoming more successful. Of course, we don't do that here; we would have to work with my colleagues at Barnes-Jewish Hospital in St. Louis. We need more information to proceed and see where we are."

A few weeks later, exploratory surgery confirmed the diagnosis through a biopsy. I looked it up, and it appeared patients were usually closer to middle age in most cases. There was no other effective treatment to "stave off" primary sclerosing cholangitis (PSC). I'd just have to make the best of it, and Dr. Greenberg would monitor the situation. St. Louis was 200 miles away but manageable given the higher level of care needed.

The diagnosis was a bit anti-climactic since this had been

going on for a year. Debby was concerned, but since I was still able and willing to live a normal life, it was hard to accept that my health was failing at such a young age. Certainly, this was something to deal with way down the road, or at least we hoped. We prioritized diet, exercise, and living as healthy while trying to live as normally as possible. We took a positive approach, expecting me to live a long life, assuming that if this progressed seriously, there was always the hope of a transplant.

Our small, two-bedroom, one-bath ranch sat on a dogleg corner of South White Street in Sidney, Illinois. Our home in a newer subdivision lacked the cool shade of the mature trees in the older parts of town. The trees on the main drag just south of the railroad tracks exploded in a brilliant display of blends of orange, yellow, and red as fall days advanced. By contrast, we had only a locust tree at the edge of our lot with minimal shade, and it sported menacing thorns, the kind that could and did flatten our riding mower tires. It also dropped dark maroon pods, giving more incentive for a chainsaw to collide with the tree's trunk.

Instead of cutting it down, I set out to fill the void of a bare lot with mail-order trees from the Henry Fields Seed & Nursery Co. But they were only four feet tall sticks. Our home was a spec house, and to keep the price down, the local contractor, Dick Mumm, did not install air conditioning. We were saving to have it installed. The home remained so hot without shade or air conditioning that we often visited our parents. At this stage of life, it was a "paycheck to paycheck" existence. Debby was staying home with the baby, as was our plan. Since I met her, she has always oriented herself toward having a husband, kids, the white picket fence, and that type of picturesque life. The trees were planted, and the family was started—but a crack of chronic illness remained in the family picture. Sickness was for the aged. But the sick bed came for me, and it came early, and no doubt changed our lives.

As the decade wore on, I completed my apprenticeship at work, which came with a moderate pay raise. Two more daughters came along with great joy—Jessica Erin, born November 2, 1985, and Rachel Caroline, born September 10, 1989.

One day, I was out walking with my oldest daughter, Ashley, who was four years old. She was playfully tossing little pebbles in a creek near our home. A friend stopped by and asked, "Do you need a ride?"

"No, thanks," I replied.

"Where are you going?"

I laughed and said, "Wherever she leads me!"

As a young father, the delight of watching a child's mind when given freedom fascinated me. I had an early life reprimand of the importance of time. With the leisure I allowed, Ashley meandered to the playground at the nearby grade school. Enjoying these activities with my kids gave me delight and helped me develop one of my best traits as a parent. Patience. Like my mother, I was naturally patient, and working with my kids helped me develop empathy to go along with being slow to anger. Not that I was a pushover. I drew firm boundaries for the kids. I did not correct them repeatedly, but rather, before my children pushed me toward anger, I sent them to their rooms to be quiet and let me know when they were ready to behave. The kids railed against this injustice, but they could fuss and cry it off in their room. Some of these principles I gleaned from Dr. James Dobson's book, *Dare to Discipline.* My parents had also been no-nonsense in their approach. You just *knew* not to push it. Debby was into teaching the kids and having educational toys to stimulate their minds. I felt we were good parents.

We checked many boxes for a successful family, but fissures developed over time.

I chalked it up to the stress of raising young children. A stay-at-home mom can feel very isolated, and I sensed this happening to Debby even before Rachel was born. After Rachel was born, Debby seemed depressed and desperate for a life change or something to shake up the day-to-day. Our conversation one day went like this, "Doug, I'm not happy, and to start with, we have outgrown this home, and I've been asking for some time what we can do?"

I heard and understood her, and she was right. I had been putting off wanting to move or build onto the home. But it was time for a change and to move us into a bigger house, whether I felt we could afford it or not.

I remained in denial about having severe marital issues. The marriage gods declared that we had a good chance at a long, happy marriage, didn't they? After all, we met *and* were married in Philo, Illinois, the "Center of the Universe," as declared by radio personality Stevie Jay. And it said so on the water tower, making it official. I later asked Stevie, now owner of his own radio stations, how it came to be.

"Our family was living in India at the time, and near the Ganges River was a structure bearing the words, 'Center of the Universe.' My older brothers concluded that if they dug straight through the earth, they would come out at Philo, Illinois! Of course, that is off geographically by three thousand miles or so." Stevie didn't let that detail get in the way of the designation for his hometown.

Seriously, though, both sets of parents had long marriages. Debby's entire family, including her aunts and uncles, had no divorces. I can't speak for Debby, but the constant workload with the kids and seeing her husband's decline becoming more visible through symptoms and jaundice must have affected her.

But I kept thinking about how our family priest, Father John Hecht of St. Thomas Catholic church, also of Philo, vetted us thoroughly and thought we were well-matched. I trusted and respected him. After our marriage, we decided to leave my Catholic and her Lutheran background for a non-denominational

Christian church in Sidney to have "our" church together and leave those of our youths behind. Father Hecht did his job, and nothing was his fault.

Religion wasn't the main problem, but I had become more serious about my faith over the years. Dying slowly or rapidly often has the effect of making a person more spiritually oriented. While Debby might have felt I went overboard with my getting involved in lay speaking for a time and more interest in ministry, she knew me well enough to know that I was too flawed and irreverent to be a leader in the church. Ask any of the guys on the work crew. I was just as into the coarse jesting and profanity as most of the guys. The witty banter and teasing of each other helped us through the inevitable monotony that comes with any job.

I thought getting a new home might keep the harmony and raise my wife's spirits. I really wanted her to be happy. The upgrade of a home was a legitimate need as well. We had these wonderful children together, and I felt we deeply bonded through shared experiences. She worked so hard with the kids in their care and learning. I thought to myself, *If we get this housing need addressed, it will be better for the children and help Debby be happier, given a more spacious home.* The decision was made to make a move.

We had our current home listed for sale, and I came home one day, and Debby was excited, "Hey honey, we have a couple interested in our house, and there is a house in St. Joseph (a nearby community) for us to look at."

I was always the more conservative financially, but seeing how excited my wife was, I was eager to look into this new home even if it stretched the budget. Men will joke about various versions of "Happy Wife, Happy Life." It's so true. The new house had three bedrooms, two full baths, an excellent school system, and was closer to work. Done deal.

We settled our young family into the attractive brick and cedar ranch home on July 4, 1990. The girls were 6 and 4, and the baby was 10 months. We had my co-workers and friends from church providing the moving help. The new, bigger home was almost palatial by the standards of what we had been used to. Would this new home provide the needed boost?

A couple of months later, I was talking at work to Mark Harms, a close friend. who was aware of our marital issues. "So, did the new house make your wife happier?"

I replied, "I wish I could say yes, but no, it is not better."

It was not better in the sense of our marriage, but actually, my wife was coming out of her depression. A friend she had recently acquired seemed to spark her imagination. One of our strengths as a couple had been that we generally shared everything pertinent to our relationship with each other. She readily admitted that the attention from this outside party made her feel better about herself. She saw possibilities to return to the workforce, which given the circumstances of my potential early disability or passing, seemed wise.

As February of 1991 came around, I celebrated my 31st birthday on the 13th and also presented my wife with a dozen beautiful roses for Valentine's Day. While well-intended, it was met with the need for a "talk." When the kids were all napping, we sat down, and Debby said, "Doug, I think you know this is not working out. This new job and new friends are important to me." She continued, "I know your illness is getting worse, and you will need this transplant soon. I just don't love you like I did before. I don't plan to leave until after you get through your surgery."

There it was. This is where I stood. I've been bucked off a horse, and that hurt, but I'd never been kicked. This was what I imagined a kick felt like. She had been dropping hints all along. Now she had come out and said it. Our family was going to split. Initially, I became angry at her new life and fulfillment outside the home. "There is no one to blame," she said. "I'm at a point in my life where I just really need to change what I'm doing. Our marriage just isn't working out."

I kept the groveling mild to moderate, as I could tell she had resolved to make a change. I wanted to say, "Oh great, you're worried about trying to make yourself happy, and I'm just trying to freaking stay alive. I'm sorry to inconvenience your departure by needing a life-saving surgery!" Rather than saying that, though, I acted in passive-aggressive ways. One night, she returned from work late and was exhausted. She just wanted to crash. My anxiety was legitimately high, but to be as annoying as possible, I brought a brown paper bag to bed and was hyperventilating. Noisily the bag inflated and deflated, and she finally departed to the couch, and I could hear faint cursing as she left the room. Was that my idea of a victory? I don't know. I just know I was stressed and anxious about everything, and I wanted to share it!

By late March, I was no longer able to work. Dr. Greenberg wanted an endoscopy to evaluate the progression of the PSC. He was concerned about varices, another curse of liver disease. In late March, while doing the endoscopy, gastric varices burst, and this caused life-threatening bleeding. I was sedated and only partially heard the stir. Dr. Greenberg calmly gave instructions. The raised voices of the nurses indicated to me as to the severity of the situation. Liver failure also inhibited my ability to stop bleeding. I was in danger of bleeding to death. I was sent back in to deeper sedation as they worked on me.

"Mr. Swinford, your children are here to see you before you take a little helicopter ride to St. Louis." Dr. Greenberg appeared and explained, "Doug, I'm sorry but your disease has caused you to have these enlarged and vulnerable veins in your stomach. One such vein burst during exam. We have it stopped and are airlifting you to Barnes-Jewish for evaluation for transplant. There isn't anything else we can do here."

After that, the kids, ages seven, five, and 18 months,

approached me, and I joked around with them with this little suction device that I had. Debby was distant, staying back with her new girlfriend, who was also going through a divorce.

After my brief visit with the kids, I was whisked into the chopper for the 200-mile ride from Central Illinois to the "Gateway to the West."

Dr. Wallis Marsh was head of the Liver Transplant team at Barnes, in March of 1991. He was upbeat as he and his group of white coated interns examined me and gathered around. "Mr. Swinford, your liver disease has advanced to the point that we are evaluating you for a transplant. We are trying to stabilize this bleeding episode. It helps that you are young, your kidney function is good, and your blood type is favorable to get a match."

I was encouraged by his words, but I sure felt terrible. Later that evening, with my parents and sister both visiting, my mom and I were happy to see them bring me some real food. I was getting lasagna, salad, and bread. My Dad and sister Debbie had stepped out. I just started eating, and my mom was putting more butter on my garlic bread. After a few bites, I felt sick and I had time for Mom to grab a basin, and here came the blood. My sister had just returned to the room, saw what happened, and ran for the nurse yelling for help.

To witness firsthand blood flowing freely out of my body meant only one thing to me–death. The bleeding episodes were survivable for one reason. They happened while in the hospital, where help was readily available.

Somehow, the bleeding situations were compensated with transfusions, and I was stabilized and able to do the evaluation. Two weeks after all the drama, I was sent home to rest and not do any lifting or anything that could cause me to start bleeding again. I did just that, and word came in early April that I was officially on the list for transplant.

It was now a waiting game. The kids buoyed me. They seemed so sensitive to my sickness. I explained everything the best that I could to them. "Girls, I need a big operation, and I will be okay." They seemed to accept this. Transplants are ironic in that I was dying, and for liver transplants, someone else had to die to give me a chance. My spirits stayed positive. I was in a very high mortality rate and was actually relishing every day as it was. I was able to keep in the background that my wife was leaving.

My friend David Vineyard, whom I met at Sidney Christian Church, chipped in and helped around the house with the kids and mowing the yard. He seemed moved by my circumstances and assisted with work that I couldn't do and also as a sounding board, all the while helping his dad run a major seed corn operation.

On June 21, 1991, I felt a little better and was outside running the weed eater. It felt good to be able to do something productive. My chores mainly consisted of keeping the kids fed and the house picked up. As life related to my spouse, I felt a deep sense of betrayal. Love or love not, I needed a friend.

Besides being my spouse, she had been my confidante for almost half my life. Every major event we went through together. I was 17, and Debby was 16 when we met. Except for a few minor breakups before marriage, we went through all of our major life events together. Her brother Denny had passed away in a pick-up truck accident in which he was a passenger when we first started dating. The loss was devastating for her and her family, and I was badly shaken as well. Other bonding-type experiences were our wedding, the difficult pregnancies, and the birth of our children. These connections forged life-long memories.

With our history, who gave a damn about Love at this point? The Tina Turner song came to mind. She sang, "What's love, got to do, got to do with it? What's love but a secondhand emotion?" I concluded that I wasn't going to understand what Debby was feeling.

The closest I came to an understanding was when I talked to my counselor, the Rev. Ralph Deal, who led seminars for people going through breakups. He explained that, for whatever reason, in his words, "People feel like they are going to explode if they don't change their circumstances."

Okay, fair enough. Debby was 30 years old and maybe felt life was passing her by. Perhaps she was intimidated by my advancing disease seeming to make its move rapidly and could find herself alone with three kids and no career. She didn't try to explain it, but one comment didn't set well with me. This was before she told me it was "over." I had an objection to something she wanted to purchase, and she said, "So are we just going to use all of our money to pay medical bills?"

Yes, having this type of illness can be devastating financially. To me, it was just another aspect of feeling like I was a liability, burden, and hassle through no fault of my own. In the period since she had given me the news that it was over in February, I had decided that I needed a plan. By June 21, I had concluded that I was going to try to convince her to go ahead and change her life, but don't disrupt mine and the kids. Let them stay in the same home with the same friends and the same school. She could have all the visitation she wanted, just please let the kids stay in their world. That was the plan I was trying to sell.

Later that evening, Friday, June 21, 1991, I had the house all picked up, dishes done, and kids were asleep. I had been listening to St. Louis Cardinals baseball playing the San Diego Padres. My city of hope was also where my favorite baseball team was located. For at least a few hours, I had put life's woes to the side. I had a good day, and I felt optimistic about the future. Their mom was still living at home and had not come home from work. I didn't know where she was and had become used to her keeping an irregular schedule. Working in real estate sometimes involved long hours, and I didn't question her. There were no cell phones in those days, so she was carrying a pager if I had an urgent need.

After the ballgame, I was watching TV when a call came in.

"Mr. Swinford, I am calling from the transplant office, and we have a liver for you. We know you live some distance away, and we would like you to be here before 3 a.m. Are you ready to go through with this?"

My heart raced, and I said, "Yes, we will get right down!" Wow, this was really going to happen! I paged Debby and woke the kids to briefly explain what was happening. They were too young to comprehend, but I did choke up thinking I might never see them again. I told them everything would be okay, and I really felt like our journey together was not over. My friend David and our Pastor Jim were on call to take me to St. Louis, but I needed their mom to come home and be with the kids. She never answered the pager.

Chapter 3

God, Can I Get a Contract Extension?

"Don't worry about it. My mother-in-law is coming quickly, and then we can go," I said.

David started to say something but held his tongue because our preacher and friend Jim Lane had come along. It was more out of respect for Jim than anything. David rarely cursed but was quite exasperated at the situation, given the importance of me getting on the road promptly. He was a hard-driving business guy, and his task appeared to be delayed.

I didn't have time to worry about where Debby had gone. It was time to go and get a job done. I felt bad for Norma, Debby's mother, who did not care to go out at night, and I had most certainly pulled her out of bed. But she pulled up within a short time.

"Helloooo," she said with enthusiasm as she came in." She always spoke almost like she was singing. "I'll see to the kids. Good luck, Doug!"

"Okay, Norma, thanks so much for coming quickly. We are off!"

I remained in a defensive mode for Debby. I would not have liked it if David had said something critical. I *married* her. If not for her, I probably would have wrapped my speedy Mustang around a tree with my foolhardy drinking. Yes, life changed, and we didn't feel the same anymore, but she was the mother of our children. She nudged me to settle down and start a family. *She* helped me create the life I had. I could be disappointed, even angry with her. Being dumped could also offer motivation. My thoughts were, *She thinks I'm going to die or be disabled. Don't you dare give up! Get well. Have a good life with or without her!*

Treatment for liver failure only existed for a brief speck of time in human history. Medical professionals made initial efforts in the late 50s and early 60s by practicing liver transplants on dogs. Dr. Thomas Starzl, known as the "father of transplantation," worked out the method to successfully remove and sew in a new liver. New and exciting surgeries began saving lives in kidney transplants as success was found in identical twins able to share a kidney that the body would not reject. It would always be the case that the closer a person was related, the more the need for suppression declined. Finding a balance of immune suppression played a key role, as early attempts with radiation were not successful. Left unchecked, the immune system would destroy the organ of an unrelated donor within a few days. Too much radiation made the patient generally ill and susceptible to infection. But some achievements started being found in a combination of the drugs Imuran and Prednisone. Dr. Starzl performed a mother-to-son kidney transplant in 1962, and the use of the new suppression cocktail gave great hope as the boy soon returned to school and normal life. This triumph led to a series of kidney transplants in which the immune suppression duo showed consistent effectiveness. Dr. Starzl's team began to show great promise that liver transplants may become feasible.

Bennie Solis, the son of Spanish-American parents, had been born with a tragic liver disease. At three years old and seriously ill, he was seen by Dr. Starzl in February 1963. At the time, there was no treatment and no precedence for liver transplantation to try and help this boy. Sure, there had been experiments done on animals. Kidney transplants had been successful, but a new kidney was sewn in, and the old organs left in place.

Liver replacement required the whole organ to be removed and a new liver sewn in—all the while keeping the patient's blood flowing to the rest of the body. Dr. Starzl and his team at the University of Colorado received the go-ahead to try and save the boy's life by performing a transplant from a young heart patient who had not survived his surgery and was on life support.

Sadly, they lost Bennie on the operating table as the bleeding was uncontrollable. The surgeons sat in the operating room for a long time and stared at the floor. It was devastating. Further attempts at liver transplant in 1963 saw patients able to survive the surgery but living just a few days or weeks. Despite the results, monumental steps had been made, and the main problems were now better defined.

In his memoir, *Puzzle People,* Dr. Starzl describes the painstaking work to further the process and how improvements started coming into practice. In 1967 he performed the first successful liver transplant and moved this monumental achievement from experimental treatment to a therapeutic reality by the early 1980s.

A patient like me with severe liver disease in 1984 had a treatment option, and from the time Dr. Greenberg diagnosed me, we knew transplant surgery was my best hope. On June 21, 1991, my bad luck of having PSC and liver failure coincided with the good luck that these brilliant medical advancements gave me a chance to prolong my life. The science for changing out the current liver for a different liver was still evolving, and techniques improved constantly.

To that end, my support team and I headed out late that night on the first day of summer 1991 to be a part of the grand experiment built on Dr. Starzl kicking the door open just 24 years prior.

If I survived this attempt to restore my emaciated and broken-down body, I felt it was a win for me and all ailing liver patients—a small victory for humanity. The misfortune of one (the donor) could help others avoid the whims of disease. Like a daffodil lying dormant under the frozen ground of winter, patients wait for spring via the transfer of life from fellow travelers who met an untimely end. The healthy organs acted as the warmth and sun to bring forth the beauty and color of life the sick once enjoyed.

As I was hoping spring would come, I settled in my room with my transport team. Pastor Jim said a prayer. "Dear God, please bring Doug through this by your power, and bless the medical people who help him; in Jesus' name, Amen." And he and David were off, as my parents and sister, Cheryl, had arrived, cutting short their attendance at my cousin Tab Gerstner's wedding in Kansas City to come to support me. I had asked permission from the transplant office to attend said wedding myself.

"Doug, that would not be a good idea. If we get a call or you have a setback, you would be too far away."

"I'll stay home. The Gerstners have great wedding parties, but it is a big family, so I'll make the next one!"

"Hey, Douglas, how are you doing?" my dad asked excitedly. My mom, dad, and sister were all ecstatic as they came into my room. It didn't matter that it was near 3:00 a.m. We were all running on adrenaline, and the staff also seemed enthusiastic. The lighting shone softly, and the room smelled clean. I could also smell coffee, the lifeblood of nurses pulling night shifts. The nurse came in with instructions for me.

"Mr. Swinford, here is a bottle of an antibacterial solution. I want you to wash your whole body with it." She gave a little demonstration, reminding me of a flight attendant with pre-flight instructions.

"Okay, I'll be sure to wash behind my ears too!"

After my shower, we visited animatedly, and time passed quickly. Suddenly, the time to go came.

"Best of luck, brother. I'm praying for you," my sister Cheryl said.

My mom and dad said, "We will see you later. Go get well."

The medical team wheeled me into the operating room at 6:00 a.m. In my mind, I thought to myself, *You have to survive! You have three little girls waiting for you and depending on you! Surely there could be a better time to die.*

As if returning from a long celestial trip, when the great fog of anesthesia lifted, I woke up in recovery nearly 13 hours later. Between my excitement at realizing that I survived to the euphoria of drugs, I felt a high I'd never previously experienced.

"Mr. Swinford, while you may not feel it yet, we will try to stay ahead of the pain that will come," the nurse said. "We are keeping you intubated, as we may have to take you back into surgery for a little leak patch-up."

I motioned for a pad and scribbled some questions about how I was doing and so forth.

"Mr. Swinford, you came through the surgery very well. You are doing great. We will get this leaky vessel fixed."

I next woke up early June 23, no more vent. Like most major

surgery patients, I had multiple drains, including an uncomfortable nasogastric tube down my nose to drain my stomach. The pain came in over the firewall to singe my nerves over the next few days.

My left arm swelled up and hurt from my shoulder to my hand. My belly felt a general throbbing. When the surgical team made their rounds, I asked Dr. Marsh, "Why does my arm hurt so bad?"

"Well, Doug, in order to do this surgery, we have to run a bypass from your upper arm to your groin to manage the blood flow." Dr. Marsh liked to add levity to the situation and also added, "Your abdominal incision won't let you down. It is going to hurt, too. It just hasn't gotten around to it yet!"

Dr. Marsh adamantly told me that this transplant was to put me back to full health and life. That was the expectation.

After the next few weeks, we dealt with a rejection episode, which resulted in me changing my medication from Cyclosporine, the standard treatment of the day, to the experimental drug named FK-506. This new drug showed superior prevention of rejection of the new organ. Prior to this drug, patients rejected their new organ when their natural immune response damaged the new organ and thus required another donor and surgery. To my benefit, this drug, while not yet FDA-approved, was available to help patients with severe rejection.

After the initial surgery and some touchy moments over the

first three weeks, I was finally able to eat a normal meal again. This was no small matter to me. Due to concerns about internal bleeding, I survived only on liquids with no solid food for several weeks. "How do you feel today, Doug?" Dr. Marsh would ask on rounds.

"I'm starving. I'm so hungry. could I maybe get even some gruel?" I said lightheartedly. "Can I have anything but broth?"

"Not yet. We are going to start an IV feeding tube to get you some protein and energy. We aren't quite sure about your digestive system yet," Dr. Marsh explained.

"Okay, I'll stop watching TV commercials with pizza and chicken and all manner of food. I can smell it when someone has bagels at the nurse's station. I'm going to make up for this when I feel better!"

When that first meal came, it was a Thanksgiving-style turkey and dressing. Right as my food came in, the Chaplain, Don, who had stayed steady with me, arrived to talk. I savored every bite and ate slowly. I met Don in one of my pre-transplant meetings, and we hit it off. He asked me to think about if I would want him to go through the surgery with me in the operating room, offering up prayers and support. "Sure, Don, I'll take all the help I can get!"

As I finished my meal, I broached the topic of the surgery for the first time.

"Don, tell me, what was it like in the operating room?"

Don looked down at the floor. The recollection seemed to

upset him. "It was hard to observe, Doug. The condition of your liver and the stress on the vessels was so intense. The surgeons had to work so delicately. It is traumatic for a layperson to watch. It is tough to see a positive outcome in the midst of all of that blood loss. The team was very composed and confident while discussing the troubles along the way."

"Don, I am so thankful for you being there. It was important for me to know you were there. It was quite a sacrifice for you to spend that much time to help me," I said earnestly.

Don, a retired minister, said, "It was my privilege, Doug, and to see that you are recovering now makes me feel good." Don glanced at the empty chair next to my bed where a spouse would usually sit.

The *empty chair* issue no longer came up in discussion after I was asked a couple of times, "Where is your wife?" I didn't even perceive at the time that maybe they had introduced me to Don as a means of support due to my marital woes. The spouses of other patients on the floor barely left the side of their loved ones during their surgery and recovery. My sister Debbie came to visit and posted a picture of my daughters that she had made into a poster, which was prominent on my wall. I didn't think about the *empty chair* when I gazed at my wonderful kids.

As regular nourishment bolstered my strength, I began to feel alive again. Dr. Marsh explained, "Doug, in your wait for a donor, your body broke down considerably. The rebuild to do the surgery was hard and has prolonged your recovery. Our hope all along has been to make an old man out of you. It is your obligation to take your medicines, keep your appointments, and be vigilant to any problems that arise. You will have to skip the cocktail hour, but you can do anything else you want, and we will see you in about six months. Then we'll discuss if you can return to work. Just don't try running any marathons yet!"

Although still slow moving and in recovery, I was discharged to return home after five weeks. As they had done 31 years ago, my mom and dad brought me home from the hospital. My parents were so wonderful. I faced a long road to recovery as my primary focus while also dealing with a divorce and a new family situation. I wanted to prove to Debby that I would recover more than ever. I would go to the gym and make myself a fitter and stronger man. Debby's rejection provided a voice in my ear, saying, *You are done and not worth waiting for.*

My reply to the inner critic was, *I guess we will see about that!*

I was still in the game. But I wondered if I would recuperate enough to return to a job that required construction work. With a divorce pending, what would my life look like afterward? Was there any chance the children could continue living with me? The division of assets was not a major concern because we had little in the way of cash, just some little equity in the house. Those were things on my mind as my parents and I rolled down the road toward my parent's home.

After all the time indoors, I was struck by the beauty of the outdoors, the lush green grass, the full trees, and the vibrant corn fields of the Midwestern landscape. I also sensed the relief that my parents felt. It looked like their boy was going to make it.

Chapter 4

Home Not So Sweet Home

After a few days of resting at my mom and dad's home to prepare for being around the kids, my sister Cheryl took me home. Debby and the kids were out, but I had a house key and rejoiced to enter our living room and sit in my recliner. The familiarity of home was a magical elixir to me. It felt so good.

Soon to follow, the kids arrived home, exclaiming, "Dad, Dad!" as they came to me. It was a joyous reunion.

Debby said rather flatly, "We didn't know you were coming."

I replied, "I'm so happy to be home. It feels so good." I observed that perhaps Debby thought I would be staying at my parents' home more permanently as a means of separation, but I had no such intentions and didn't feel I needed an invitation to come to my own home. My sister Cheryl, sensing the tension, said her goodbyes to all and left.

"Girls, you need to pack your bags. We need to go," Debby said.

The kids were noticeably puzzled and became tearful but complied. Both my body and mind felt too weak and stunned to mount any inquiry about where they were going or why. But within about 45 minutes of finally being home, I sat alone in my quiet house.

I sat and collected my thoughts. I didn't turn the television on or play any music in the aftermath. I felt surprised by what had transpired, trying to grasp everything that had happened throughout the weeks leading up to this abandonment. What I did know was that life had made a dramatic change. My anatomy underwent alteration and required special care for the rest of my life. My almost ten-year marriage was over, but the details around our separation remained unresolved. The unknowns in that realm troubled me more than anything. It had taken time for all of these events to come together, both the good and the bad. However, the application of time and patience remained the only remedy to my travails.

I heard the garage door open an hour after Debby and the kids left. The kids walked in with their bags in hand and calmly took their stuff to their rooms. Ashley and Jessica helped Rachel with her bags since she was not quite two years old. Debby came in briefly, but we didn't talk, and she spoke with the girls and then left. I didn't register it then, but this was our official separation. While we saw her from time to time, she no longer lived with us and gradually took her possessions bit by bit.

I'd be remiss if I didn't admit to having a slight hope of reconciliation after getting through the big surgery. Perhaps I was still kind of high on the pain medications, but in speaking with Debby's parents on the phone two days post-surgery, I said, "I think it will all work out, and we can fix our problems now that I'm getting better."

Debby's parents, the late Bill and Norma, were happy too. Bill said, "Get better, Doug, and we will see you soon!"

I also told my friend David over the phone, "Dave, I think since I have come through this that Debby and I can work it out."

David remained dubious but supportive and said, "Well, we will see how it all works out but keep your expectations reasonable."

He was right, but I was in the manner of thinking to myself, *Hey, you survived this. All things are possible.* I was in denial, assisted by narcotics. However, as the rawness of the pain and the clearing of the mind caught up with me, I accepted the reality of the relationship not being viable.

After bringing the girls back home, their mom departed, and a sense of tranquility set in. Debby and I hadn't been arguing or yelling at each other, but the tension had been palpable. Now we were moving on. I needed to focus on trying to recover my health, and she was trying to rebuild her life and get healthy from her disappointment with how life was going. She had the desperate need to seek fulfillment by other means; by now, I was on board with that. I repeated in my discussions with her, "Debby, I understand your need to change your life. Please allow the kids and I to keep life as similar as possible regarding school, friends, and the home." I believed this with all of my heart.

Of course, we each sought legal counsel, and the custody being up in the air caused me tremendous stress. I couldn't imagine being outside looking in at my kids' lives. Worse yet, if she were to remarry and the kids were living under the roof of a stepdad. I could not imagine a scenario where moving to another town and being under different circumstances would be for their benefit. The kids and I were close and getting closer now that I was their primary caregiver.

Despite my confidence being shaken in the aspects of ego, self-esteem, ability to work, and moving on to any future relationships, I believed in my parenting ability. I had the potential to develop my mother's patience. I loved being a dad. I was probably a better dad than a husband, as I may have missed opportunities to support my wife. I knew she was down sometimes, but I didn't know what to do to help her. As it stood now, the kids needed extra support for the transitions that divorce would take us through, and I was fortunate that my period of disability allowed me to be a full-time dad.

As part of my recovery, the kids and I took walks down our sidewalk, sometimes to the nearby Hackler Park. On one of these walks, I stopped to visit with a neighbor, and he asked, "Do you mind if I ask how you are making a living?" He could tell I was at home full-time.

I took no offense to the question and said, "Gordy, I have sick leave from my job, and I also qualified for Social Security Disability. We don't make near what we were, but we are able to get by." I continued, "Gordy, you might be surprised too, but my co-workers, spearheaded by Wilbur Clark, did a fundraiser for me, raffled off a hog, and gave us the proceeds. As it turns out, some of the raffle ticket buyers put our name on their ticket, so besides the monies, we also won half a hog!"

While we were starting to transition to a new church in our new town of St. Joseph, we also received a generous collection taken at our previous church, the Sidney Christian Church. "Gordy, people have been very generous to us, and we truly hope to keep the house." He seemed very gratified to hear that we were getting along okay and had received such gifts.

Friends warned me that I was going to get wiped out financially by the divorce. That was impossible as we didn't have enough assets to squabble over. Yes, I had to borrow money from my dad to pay Debby half of the house's equity, which was under ten thousand dollars. We were a young couple with three kids and hadn't saved much. The real issue was the custody. "Debby, please do what you need to and visit anytime you want, but don't shake up the kids' world."

Debby said, "If we have a joint agreement, I need visitation rights most anytime, with reasonable notice, of course."

I said, "I will do everything to help with any and all visitation, and the kids can call anytime as well. I give you my promise that I won't stand in the way of any request. And even if you want a few days here and there, it can be arranged." I was serious, too, and had full intentions of keeping my word.

There was no dramatic court scene of fighting over the children. I'm not implying in any way that we never exchanged harsh words about custody. Divorce makes for tension and grating conversations. One day on the phone, I told Debby with a raised voice, "I will fight in court for joint custody and to keep the kids living with me. I don't care what it costs!"

Debby barked back, "Well, you have heard of parents just taking off with their kids, and the other parent never sees them again?"

I'm not sure who hung up first, but the conversation ended abruptly. What she said concerned me, but I knew she wouldn't do anything like that.

Pragmatism ruled the day. Debby consulted with her lawyer, and we scheduled a meeting with counsel to avoid court, and it was all settled. "Joint" custody with me having physical custody, and she had every other weekend and any other time requested. With that settled, I secured a sense of stability in the household. I'm forever grateful that Debby made this decision, which I believe was made solely in the girls' best interest. Neither of us entertained contemplations about what others might say. Any gossip or whispers about our divorce or custody were topics that I'm sure lost their flavor very quickly, and the next misfortune someone had would be more interesting fodder.

The girls and I could settle in, let the rest of the divorce proceedings work their course, and move on with life. Jessica was five and starting kindergarten, and her little sister Rachel and I were allowed to go in and listen to the teacher introduce the kids to school while I recorded a video. I could abide the pain that still accompanied me from surgery. I wouldn't miss this first school day moment for anything. The kids continued thriving regardless of my body being a badly bruised vessel. But my spirits were up, and we looked ahead to a bright future.

Chapter 5

Werewolf Blues

After I had cleared the bar to get placed on the transplant list and was being prepared for "life after transplant," I had been required to travel to the clinic in St. Louis for a series of meetings in the late weeks of May 1991.

The meetings consisted of talking with a social worker and a discussion with my transplant coordinator. The social worker discussed who would help take care of me at home and asked if I had adequate emotional support. I was forthcoming about my tenuous marital situation, which was not ideal. However, it did not disqualify me from the transplant since I had other family and friend support. And no doubt, with this being an expensive proposition, the conversation led to insurance and financial talks. Fortunately, I had decent health insurance, and my transplant was covered, which most insurance companies have covered as therapeutic since the early 1980s. There were payment plans for what insurance didn't cover. Though limited, my steady income was enough to make it work. Sick pay was partial pay, but at least I *had* sick pay.

Most compelling to me was the visit with the liver transplant coordinator. We had become quite well acquainted since my initial visit in March. Debbie Sutter said, "Now, Doug, your immune suppression is the most critical item in what will be a long med list." She emphasized her point, adding, "You *have* to take this medicine *for the rest of your life*. Along that line, I need to know if you want to participate in a clinical trial for a new therapy that is not yet FDA-approved. This new drug is showing promise in preventing rejection. After we get you through surgery, we have to slow down your immune response. Cyclosporine is our primary form of treatment, but the experimental FK-506 is in trials. Our staff needs to know if you wish to take part in this study?"

I had read about this FK-506 and how it was showing superior results over the standard treatment to preserve organs. "Yes, I'd like to take it," I said.

Debbie replied, "Well, we can't assign you the medicine. There are protocols, and you have to draw an envelope, and you will get either the standard treatment or the experimental treatment."

"Okay, fair enough."

I pulled an envelope out of a basket, and it designated me to start on the standard of cyclosporine. I felt the FK-506 was outperforming the standard and would have helped my chances. It was also free during the trial period, which would have been very helpful.

With that resolved, my coordinator then went on at length about the risks of taking immune suppression drugs and how careful I would need to be to prevent infection. All forms of bacteria, viruses, and fungi could try and take advantage of my weakened immune system. This was part of the risk. My body would see that this new organ didn't have the "password" to my system. It was an invader that needed to be destroyed. And with that, the suppression actually knocked out some of the good T cells. To curb this, prednisone was added to the long list, which, as one of the doctors described with a laugh, "Makes the immune response act like a person who had a few beers."

One final thing, discussed almost as thoroughly as the suppression, was the need to hydrate the kidneys. Immune suppressants were somewhat toxic to the kidneys. In Ms. Sutter's words, "The suppression therapy is going to pound your kidneys!" She pounded her fist into her palm. "It is essential that you drink a lot of water every day to help maintain good kidney function."

I told her that I would do so. I was thinking, *This is a lot to take in. Sure, this isn't going to be easy. It is life-saving and life-altering at the same time.*

Since I was already in St. Louis for the day, I stayed for the transplant support group meeting that evening. I didn't know anyone who had received a liver transplant. In the meeting, I met several people on the list like me, but I was impressed with the recipients that were there and how healthy they looked. They looked *normal.* What did I expect? I asked a woman around my age how she was doing. She said, "It has been challenging, but I feel really good now at a year out. You can do this, too. Just be patient. Most of us have found that you have to roll with the punches." She continued, "Most of us have learned to not get too high or too low." I thanked her. Beforehand, I had doubts about whether it would be worth staying for the meeting but afterward felt grateful for the information gained.

And with the advice and education I had received, I was as ready as could be when the call came on June 21, 1991.

Living with a transplant started a little rocky for me. I was easing into the first week with the new gift when I received the news that I was going into rejection. I had drawn cyclosporine, and so far, my immune system wasn't having it. My immune system was doing what it was programmed to do: fighting invaders. The medicine also made my skin feel very oily. The surgeon, Dr. E. Steven Woodle, came in and explained, "Doug, you may not be able to tell, but you are having a significant rejection episode. You have started with cyclosporine, and we have a protocol for you to be able to change to FK-506. I'm going to try to speak to regulators to waive the lengthy process to change because we don't want to risk losing this liver."

In a unique circumstance and with my rabbit ears, I overheard the doctor make *the* call at the nurses' desk to try to get me changed over to FK-506. I deduced that he was questioned about following the protocol. "We could lose this patient or have to try and re-transplant him. We *really* need some flexibility here. I haven't lost any organs with patients using FK-506!" I could only imagine his frustration with the long, tedious surgery and seeing my immune system rallying over cyclosporine. A tech came into the room to check my blood pressure, so I didn't hear it all. What I heard, though, was Dr. E. Steven Woodle fought for me. He leaned in the room, looked at me, and gave a thumbs-up.

In getting this complex surgery, I was now part of the ongoing process to hone liver transplantation and to take part in the trial and effectiveness of FK-506. Was it really superior? What were the side effects? The disclaimer I signed to start the drug had a list of possible side- effects, including death, because there wasn't enough known about it. My two primary nurses, Ted and Misty, were in the room that day when they brought my first dose. Ted exclaimed in a serious voice, "We don't know what this will do to you; for all we know, you might turn into a werewolf!"

I grabbed my pillow to splint myself as I started chuckling. Misty turned away to cover her laugh and scolded Ted, "Come on, Ted, you can't say things like that!" I loved it, though. And who knows, maybe I could transform into a werewolf. I certainly felt like howling at times for some of the pain. To cope with Ted's mentioned risks, I would monitor my conduct at the full moon and report myself if I felt inclined to bite anyone!

The initiation in the transplant club started unsteady, but the experimental drug pulled me right out of rejection. I was headed home a little over a month after my June 22 surgery.

"Dad, what are all of those pills for?" my oldest daughter Ashley inquired.

I sat all three girls down and filled them in. "These pills are very important, and I must take them daily. If I drop or leave anything open, you are not to take any of these pills, and you have to make sure your little sister doesn't get them, either. While they help me, they could make you girls very sick."

"But, Dad, one of those is a Tylenol?" asked Jessica.

"That's right, and I'm taking that because some of these other pills I take give me a headache."

I was referring to the FK-506, as one of the side effects was headaches. Another common effect of the higher doses required in the early stages was tremors, and I had a noticeable shake of my hands.

In the early months of post-surgery, lab work was required twice a week. This testing monitored liver and kidney function and blood counts. The level of immune suppression, called the "trough level," was also checked. Weight and blood pressure readings were required daily and then weekly after a few months. My transplant hospital was some distance away, but my lab work could be done locally at Carle Hospital, and the results faxed to St. Louis. The more stability I gained, the less oversight was required. And fewer needle sticks.

In late August 1991, after being home and stable for a month, the kids and I ventured out for our first "outing." We went to Prairie Farms in Champaign, where they had a petting zoo, and the kids had a wonderful time. When we arrived home that night, and the kids were in bed, I was undressing to take a shower, and in doing so, I inadvertently pulled on a tube the surgeons had left in my side for access to put dye into my bile ducts to make sure things were working. I thought I had the tube taped firmly, but the humidity and sweat had caused the tape securing the tubing to come loose. The tape stuck to my shorts, so when I took them off, it caused a hard pull and sharp pain in my abdomen. I managed a shower, but the pain continued and intensified. Had I pulled something loose inside?

I called my parents. "Mom, I'm sorry to bother you guys, but I'm hurting so bad, I can't move. Can you please come?"

After a brief stint in the local ER, I was sent back to St. Louis by ambulance. I quickly discovered that as a transplant patient, I was treated with kid gloves, and the medical staff were ultra-cautious in doing no harm and worked to get me to my transplant center.

The next day, Dr. Marsh came in, and with a smile, he said, "What were you in such a hurry to get your clothes off for?" His white-coated followers all had a good laugh, too, and I appreciated the humor. He was buying none of my story. "Well, Doug, by pulling so hard on that tube, it leaked bile into your general body cavity, which causes an excruciating reaction. We had to remove the tube, but you will be fine with a few days of antibiotics."

I chalked this up to the first lesson of "roll with the punches."

The details of the daily medications and regular monitoring became just a part of life. I could begin to put the major surgery behind me and look to the future. My mind would sometimes drift to if I would ever date again, and if so, how would I share my health condition? I planned a tongue-in-cheek strategy that would help take the lighter side approach. It would go like this: "Hi, my name is Doug, and I have a scar so large I've been told that it looks like I had an autopsy. This is because I had liver disease and had a transplant. The medicine I take may turn me into a werewolf. On top of that, I have three little girls at home. Do you still want to talk?" I found this humorous in a way, but really, who would want to pick through this train wreck? Then again, women were known to pick up stray cats, cads, or even tipplers from time to time. Maybe one would take pity on me. Or see some potential. I had a good job. I was well groomed. I was nice most of the time. Wouldn't that all count for something?

I was reluctant to put myself in that position, at least for a while. I acquired a female friend I had met in high school who worked at the local lab and lived nearby, so she offered to take my labs at home for me along with other shut-ins. This was a tremendous help, so I didn't have to get a babysitter all of the time. My extent of knowing her was that she had given me a ride on the back of a Yamaha 80 motorcycle in high school. At that time, she seemed shy, and we didn't really talk and went to different schools, so I didn't really see her again. Fast forward 15 years later, she was an outgoing and very attractive divorcée. It was sure nice having a woman about the age of the girl's mom helping us. The kids just loved it every time she came to the house. But hey, this was all business! She had a job to do, and it helped me out.

I was quite self-conscious of how thin I looked, and I needed to regain strength if I was ever to return to a physical job. I needed to put as much muscle on my slight frame as possible. I came in last in the family in height with my brother at 6′, and I was just below my sisters, who are both 5′8″. The muscle wasting away had been dramatic as liver failure and the inability of my body to make protein left it to scavenge. As soon as lifting restrictions came off, I would have to hit the gym.

One Saturday night in mid-September 1991, after I had been home from surgery for about two months, I had the kids to bed and was just relaxing in my easy chair and watching baseball on the television. It was a lovely and quiet summer night, and suddenly I heard a knock on the screen door. To my surprise, my helper from the lab, Penny, was at the door. "Hi, do you care if I come in?" she asked.

"No, please do. I'm just watching TV."

As she sat on the couch, she said, "My boyfriend and I had a disagreement, and I just told him to take me home. It was early, and the kids are gone to their dad's, so I thought I would see how you were doing?" I was so pleased and flattered. We had a nice conversation, and she reclined on the couch and actually fell asleep.

Being a transplant patient had brought me a friend. I didn't have to tell her about my condition; she already knew. After she fell asleep, I just placed a light blanket over her and headed to bed only to be greeted in the morning by my ever-vigilant middle daughter Jessica rapping on my bedroom door, "Dad, Dad, Penny is here."

Penny apologized for falling asleep on the couch but helped with breakfast, and the kids were so excited. I worked up my nerve, and later that week, I asked her to dinner as appreciation for her help with the lab work. She accepted, and we had a splendid date, and I kissed her and held her a bit at the end of the evening. Her kindness and attractiveness stirred me with desire, but I needed to hold back and ensure she wasn't just being polite. I was getting way out over my skis. As Aristotle said, "Nature abhors a vacuum." I had come through such chaos and tumult and felt physically, mentally, and spiritually broken. Penny was a welcome salve to my soul, and she seemed to find a sort of redemption for herself in helping me. I had the love of my children, which was now supplemented by the friendship of a beautiful, hard-working woman who was also a great mother to her two young girls, Stephanie and Stacey. From the affection we shared on the first date, I felt this could move into a romantic relationship.

"Hey, don't throw it over my head." Penny and I were pitching and catching a softball during a family trip to Crystal Lake Park in Urbana. We had all five girls with us, and Stephanie and Jessi became fast and forever friends. It was a lovely fall day; we kicked the leaves around and soaked up the color. The kids played, and we ate some lunch. Penny was athletic and played on a softball team, so she kept her arm conditioned for pitching. I was ecstatic; this was so much fun. And the kids getting along so well made me think we could make this work. Not just her and me, but all of us. Together. We could work through anything.

Freud would analyze it as my id was ready to disregard caution and jump right in while my ego flashed some yellow lights. My inner voice was trying to say, *Hey, Doug, hello! Don't you remember what just happened with your soon-to-be ex-wife?*

Id won that battle, and we began to date and developed a passionate relationship. Having been so low, I found so much comfort in our love and affection. Never a cuddly guy, I could hold Penny and feel a particular connection that I had not known before.

"Penny, you are so amazing to me. You make me believe that I can be happy again. I appreciate all the help with the girls, too; they really enjoy you."

"Doug, I feel so good being with you. I'll do everything I can to help you. I'm so attracted to how you love your kids and try and instill good values in them. I *want* to be part of your life." I was truly blessed, and it was great to have a partner as I learned how to navigate this post-transplant and post-marriage existence.

As a transplant patient in 1991, the reactions I received from friends and family were, first off, a great surprise that I survived! Next, they approached me with excitement when my eyes were no longer yellow, and I began to fill out physically again. Having seen my rail-thin, emaciated body and sallow complexion, my new healthy look was a dramatic change. The compliments helped me to believe in myself, and I was able to return to my job in January 1992.

Just so I didn't forget what had transpired, all I had to do was observe my large scar, which could be compared to a Mercedes-Benz insignia. I came to be self-conscious of the road map drawn across my abdomen. Penny insisted, "Doug, you should be proud of the scars. It represents the action taken to save you and that it came at a price." A number of stitches popped up like volunteer corn. These were sharp barbs. If it were fishing line, it would be the kind you used for deep-sea fishing. When I was back in the clinic for a check-up, I asked the doctor, "What happened here?" Without an explanation, she started clipping them off at the skin. Then she said, "Okay, Doug, I'm going to have to give you a few shots to numb up to get this other one. The stitches have done their job, and your skin has fused. You are all good."

Penny and her girls came along to church with us, and Penny was baptized and joined our church. We were both very happy. My ex-wife was skeptical, offering the advice that Penny's intentions were based on the newer ranch home we lived in and her desire to move in with us. It was an attractive but typical home for the neighborhood at just over 1,400 square feet. There was no mansion or deep pockets to be had. Besides, I had a counselor, and I had no need for my ex-wife to manage my love life.

After two years, though, and when it would seem appropriate to commit more seriously with an engagement, I started to get cold feet. My counselor, the Rev. Ralph Deal, explained, "Doug, what happened to you before with loss of ability to work, health, wife, and near loss of life made you feel so out of control. Penny is a special woman. The timing of when you started dating may have come too soon for you. Penny is a couple of years ahead of you in being single. In the long run, I think it could work out for you two."

Ralph had taught classes called "Divorce and Personal Growth" seminars. Later, he changed the name to "When Your Relationship Ends." These classes were incredibly therapeutic. Ralph did a lot of couples counseling and had tremendous insight. It was an immense asset for many people who came from miles around to attend his classes.

Ralph really liked Penny and saw why I was so drawn to her.

But I had to base my decision on what I felt at the time. I told Ralph, "How can I hold and continue a connection that I have my doubts about while she thinks we are good and growing?"

Ralph understood that. "You know, Doug, if it doesn't work out right now, being single is not only not a bad thing for you, it might be the *right* move." Ralph had a good point. I had not had a chance to be single at all. I loved being single before I married. It allowed a level of independence and would allow me to work through the raising of my kids. Without question, I *never* expected anyone to help raise my kids.

In my calculations of breaking off with Penny, my subconscious chipped in that maybe we could cool things off for a while but maintain having sex. My inner critic blasted me on that thought, *Not only are you shameful, you are stupid to even think that!*

I called my friend Kevin as I mulled this over. "Buddy, what do you think? You have known Penny a lot longer than I have." I knew I was going to get an objective assessment.

"Penny is great. First off, she's hot; she's a looker. She hasn't had the easiest path in life. Her mom would yell at her for the slightest thing–I heard it one time when we brought her home just a little late. Her dad was good to her. Her ex-husband Bill is easygoing but was a skirt chaser. She's been hurt. If you married her, you could depend on her. I know she cares for you, but if you aren't sure anymore, you need to get out and see what happens. It's not fair to string her along."

I asked Penny for a sit-down meeting. She wore a look of trepidation when she arrived at my house. We sat on the couch. "Penny, I love you and care for you very much, but I just need to back off of our relationship for now." I didn't know what else to do, but I had now deeply hurt a person who had done so much to help me through my trials and rebuild my life.

While some tears appeared, I saw a flash of anger. "Doug, I don't know why you are doing this. We are so good as a couple. Our kids get along so well. You aren't going to find anything like what we have."

I knew I was going to have to let her vent it out. I had no explanation that would help anything. As she prepared to leave, she stuck me with an effective barb. It was some version of, "You and your phony farce of a spiritual life." As she walked out, an object, perhaps a shoe, was tossed across the room. I told you she was a pitcher. As for the comments, ouch, that was a deep burn there, but what could I say?

The biggest roadblock to the whole relationship was my own insecurity. I was on cloud nine at the start. I mean, we both *believed* we had met that "soul mate." Nothing could come between us. That search for unconditional love can be so elusive.

When I started to feel a shift, I agonized over how to handle it. Eventually, her intuition would sense a change in me. The romantic stage was still there, but logic and fear had overlapped the love, and I sought to restore order and safety by eliminating risk.

After my spiel, it was never the same between us. We still tried to rekindle things a few times over the next couple of years to no avail. We evolved into one of that painful on-and-off-again experiences. It didn't have to be that way if I had broken off cleanly and stuck with it. I guess I still needed to know she was there for me. One day I was standing in my kitchen doing dishes and peering out the window. The phone rang, and Penny and I engaged in a friendly conversation. We caught up on the kids and what else was going on. When we were getting ready to end the call, Penny said the sweetest thing to me. "Doug, we will be together again someday, even if it is in the nursing home!" After four years of dating, we realized it was over, and we had peace.

I felt happy just being a single dad. The communication and closeness with the girls seemed the best when I didn't have a serious relationship. We worked together, and they had to do more in the household than most kids. Ashley and Jessi helped with their younger sister. I would have my random fevers and headaches. I would come home at times and announce, "Girls, I don't feel good this evening. I'm going to put on some mac and cheese and put out some deli turkey for sandwiches, and then I'm going to bed."

"Okay, Dad, can we get on AOL?" Ashley would connect the dialup zig-zag shriek to connect to the internet, and before long, dialogue boxes would pop up with a ring on our Macintosh. Jessi would do cartwheels in our large living room while waiting her turn, and Rachel would be at her Barbie house changing outfits and combing the hair of the dolls. The kids understood when I was down.

Otherwise, we didn't discuss the transplant stuff anymore. We had put the health thing more in the background. I didn't get out often, but the girls visited their mom every other weekend, and I would occasionally go out to a Saturday night dance. I had a significant period that I didn't date at all, and I had established a comfort level around that.

So one night in 1997, I went out to a dance. I had taken a few lessons at the local Regent Ballroom, but this was a singles dance at the Urbana Civic Center.

"Do you want to dance?" I asked a lady whom I had never met.

"Okay," she said with a smile.

Donna was a nurse. Hearing her occupation put me at ease. And again, another wonderful person and mother. Like Penny, she accepted me and my problems. She believed in me. She wasn't put off by my aging Ford Aerostar van, which hardly made for romantic dates. We enjoyed some very good times together, but the relationship was fairly short-lived. Again, I couldn't stick with it. I was able to identify her sincerity much earlier. She was such a kind and giving person in an almost saintly way. She was a better person than me. That is good in one way but can be a tad intimidating for the sake of balance. She made a quick connection with the kids. I had to protect their feelings since I was skittish when it got hot in the kitchen. My youngest daughter Rachel came to be particularly sore at me.

"Rachel, you will understand when you get older. Two people can care for each other, but that doesn't mean they will stay together forever."

Even after that disappointment, Rachel continued to try and pick up women for me, often inviting them over to our home. On an outing to putt-putt golf, I invited a female friend to meet the girls and me to try it out. We enjoyed clowning around and hitting the balls errantly. As we were leaving, Rachel suggested that the friend come to the house. Playing along, she said, "But Rachel, where would I sleep?"

Rachel was six years old and had a ready reply, "You can sleep with my dad!"

As the dating implies, I had resumed a reasonably normal life and continued to date off and on. The most fun dates were through a local daddy-daughter date night program. What a blast! No pressure, no expectations, just dress up, share some snacks, a dance or two, and most importantly, just being *together*. Generally, we took turns and went solo, but Rachel enjoyed it so much she took her friend Chrissy one year.

But in the hustle and bustle of school, work, and attending music, sports, and other school activities for the girls, the 90s went fast. I was taking night classes at Parkland College in

Champaign as well. The kids enjoyed seeing what I was learning about, and life felt normal most of the time.

The main symptoms of PSC are chills and fevers, and I had mild to moderate fevers that were a nuisance but not disabling for long periods. I wasn't sure if my symptoms indicated I was sick again or just general issues post-transplant. I had more downtime than the average person, as the fevers would run the course sometimes overnight, at other times over two or three days. Overall, we had a decent nine-year period post-transplant, and I only took a few sick days a year. But I took my list of issues to see my new doctor back at Barnes for a thorough check.

Dr. Mauricio Lisker-Melman, a gastroenterologist, was now my doctor at Barnes-Jewish Hospital. I told him of my symptoms and that Dr. Greenberg at home was concerned about a recurrence of PSC. He examined me and the results from the tests conducted before my appointment. "Doug, we have observed some compromised bile ducts. The disease is coming back and causing damage to your liver. We never know with PSC. It comes back for some patients, and for others, it does not. We can't really explain why."

As he continued to spell out the situation and troubling news, I fixed my gaze on a ubiquitous glass jar on the desk containing cotton balls. I went into a daydream recalling the delights of times shared with the kids, such as their fun at Walt Disney World in Orlando, where we made a late evening run through all the rides after the crowd had dispersed for the day. I thought back to my oldest daughter Ashley's eighth-grade graduation, and I had become so emotional that my little girl was growing up. Being there for both Jessica and Rachel's first day of school. Milestones and memories that stuck in my mind. The new loves I had found and later lost. I didn't want to absorb bad news and did not intend to disrespect Dr. Lisker. I needed to feel the highlights of the past nine years before I could give credence to what I heard and its implications.

Finally, Dr. Lisker finished his talk about the progression of the disease and said, "Doug, do you have any questions?" I flinched as I came back to reality.

He was asking a question, and I responded weakly, "Is there anything else we can do about the fevers?"

The doctor responded, "We can install a biliary drain, which will leave a tube in your side and a collection bag on the outside. It may be just temporary, but we can try it."

Yuk. I didn't like the sound of that, but I didn't care for the shaking chills that blankets could not stop, no matter how high they were piled.

With this information, I learned that living with a transplant meant I would only get a limited time despite the transplant. As I left the doctor's office, I again tried not to think about the frightful prospect of going through liver failure again. Try as I might, my subconscious cut through to one question. *How long would it be before I was on the ropes?* Any discussions of further transplants were prefaced with the difficulty and risk due to the previous work. It sounded to me as if you were going to take apart a car motor to replace a part, but instead of being able to loosen nuts and bolts, the motor was welded together. At any rate, I could mull that over on the three-hour drive home. I was looking for a little escape at the time, so I headed to the riverboat casino just across the Mighty Mississippi and into the *Land of Lincoln.*

CHAPTER 6

RUNNING FROM THE DARKNESS

I had the new diagnosis, but I just wasn't ready to take it on. I was looking for the edgier side of life, and there were plenty of vices to enjoy just over the river on the Illinois side. A riverboat casino and scattered strip clubs were close to the highway. Gambling sounded better than scantily clad pretend girlfriends, and I found myself playing blackjack. At home, I had a young lady who did home daycare for us in the summer, holding the household down so I didn't have to head right home after the day trip for the doctor's visit. My two older daughters, both in high school, were in and out with jobs and school activities most days anyway. With those bases covered, I said to myself, *Hey, what the hell? I can afford to blow a couple hundred bucks*. That was how I played when I went to the casino. I considered it entertainment, and I quit when I spent all my allotted money.

On this particular day, it was give and take at the blackjack table. The smell of cigarette smoke lingered heavily in the air, and the musical sounds of the slot machines sang in the background.

Having gone electronic payouts, I missed the clinking of the dropping coins for a good hit on the slots. Downtown Las Vegas might be the only place to play with coins anymore, but I thought it made slots or video poker more fun. I sat at the cheapest table with a $5 minimum. It was great people-watching, with some folks very aggressive with their money. I enjoyed it as we had a streak of the dealer busting his hand seven out of ten times. This allowed me to play longer with house money. I was distracted, and I put my troubles on hold. I lost track of time. It was rare that I could be away a whole day, and now I was lost in the moment.

After a couple of hours, the kids started trying to reach me. I glanced at my text messages enough to see it was nothing urgent. I told them where I was and that I would head home soon.

Since I was generally more predictable, the kids became concerned that perhaps I was in over my head with gambling. Who was the parent here? It was amusing that they would be concerned with what I was doing. We didn't have enough assets to worry about that, and I hadn't gone underwater yet at the tables. I was up as far as $125, then in the hole $40, and finished up very close to even with about $20 to the house. Pretty cheap for a couple hours of entertainment, as I had to study my play chart for when to split and double down. I played well enough to not get scolded by anyone and to have a good time, and my mind was far away from a doctor's office. An evening well spent.

The doctors had told me the clock was running out on my

stable health. Armed with that knowledge, I felt the need to make more family memories. Shortly after the diagnosis, I called a family meeting and suggested we go to Panama City Beach, Florida. My oldest daughter Ashley firmly opposed this idea.

"Dad, that sounds so boring. Why don't we go back to Disney World?"

I had a quick answer to that. "Ashley, if you will recall, the last time we went to Orlando, all you girls wanted to do was go to the water parks. Especially the wave pool. Why don't we go see some real waves and enjoy the sandy beach?"

Ashley knew I valued her opinion, and she gradually came around but still felt it was a second-rate plan.

I booked a hotel right on the beach. The waves rolled in as the invisible pull of the moon regulated the tide. No, we didn't have the bright blue and higher waves of the Pacific, but the Atlantic still provided a dramatic view for us in contrast to our usual scenery of fields of corn, beans, and wheat and the livestock farms that dotted Central Illinois.

Once we arrived, the kids started having fun immediately. After a long day at the hotel pool, Jessica lobbied, "Dad, you just have to let Ashley stay down at the pool for another hour with the boy from Texas!" Jessica made a passionate plea for her older sister.

"No, no, and no," I said. I was quite familiar with what goes on in the mind of a teenage boy. "She's coming up with us to the room. Besides, we have been down here all day."

Turns out, the real action remained at the hotel pool. Ashley, who had argued against the trip, spent almost all her time talking with this boy and hanging out in the pool. Jessica enjoyed visiting with any and all of the other guests while keeping a close eye on her sister and her crush. Rachel, the youngest, rarely got out of the water and was content to play with other kids or just herself. My job was to keep the kids fed, and a Pizza Hut outlet at the pool proved the most convenient. We had a delightful time. However, the stop on the way home at the National Naval Aviation Museum at Pensacola was met with skepticism.

"Come on, Dad, it's just a bunch of old airplanes!"

And in the pictures we took at the museum, the girls are mocking enjoyment in posing by the planes. But I got to see something that *I* wanted to see.

Another added bonus: we soon found magic in looking back at the pictures. even though the kids weren't interested in the beautiful planes and careful displays, they cherish that we went there.

In the fall of 2000, after our Florida trip, my company offered me the chance for a full-time crew leader position. There was a caveat. I had to report to Danville 22 miles away instead of the 10 miles to Urbana.

I accepted the job, and my long-time friend Harry Mills and I worked the crew to cover Danville, Tilton, Georgetown, and

Ridge Farm. These were towns down Route 1, south of Danville, all tucked in the far east side of Illinois, very close to the border with Indiana. The area had been struggling economically since the closing of the General Motors Foundry in 1996, and several other high-paying companies left town. At any rate, I received a significant pay raise, and Harry and I were both baseball fans and got along well.

On a job right after the New Year, we were working in conjunction with the water company. My co-worker, Jesse Driver, and one of the water company guys hatched a plot to have me and a female employee of the water company meet.

"Sure, why not?" I said when asked if I wanted to meet her. I was told that she was 29, had two young daughters, and was a very hard worker. I was getting close to my 41st birthday, and my girls were growing up. But I loved kids, and her having kids didn't lessen my interest. After the job was complete, we headed to downtown Danville where the water company guys told us to go. Melisa worked in the area, reading meters. I rolled out of the truck to say hi to her. I had my Carhartt overalls on, and my hair was all mussed from my hard hat.

She approached us, and I quickly introduced myself. "Hi, my name is Doug Swinford. Nice to meet you."

She responded with a shy smile and said, "Hi, I'm Melisa."

Given that I was no longer a tenderfoot in dating, I wasted no time. "Would you like to go to an REO Speedwagon concert with me in a few weeks?"

"I think I'm free," she said. "We can exchange numbers, and I'll let you know."

I thought to myself, *Okay, that was a good sign. She didn't tell me to drop dead or that she had to wax her cat.*

Cute and petite, and I liked the way Melisa carried herself. The endorsement by co-workers was refreshing. My experience was that a woman working in a male-dominated field was judged harsher by her fellow workers. But all I heard about Melisa was that she divorced about a year prior, came from Indiana, and was a good person and hard worker.

I was coming into a phase with my girls where I was getting more freedom. My oldest daughter Ashley would graduate high school soon and be off to college, and Jessica wasn't far behind.

It didn't take long before I was smitten with Melisa. Despite her occupation and working in the field, she was immensely feminine. She was pretty alluring when she put her hair up while working on a ladder painting a room at home. She possessed the charm of a small-town Indiana girl.

Logistics were a problem, though. At that time, my girls had the attitude of, "Whatever makes you happy, Dad." Rachel enjoyed it when Melisa's girls were around. She was in the late part of middle school, and high school beckoned. After all of my caution in my previous relationships, I threw caution to the wind in this case. I was well aware that I likely didn't have 30 or 40 years. Hell, I might not live five years. So I felt a bit of urgency to get on with life and give up the dating thing. We could make a good team.

I warned Melisa early in our relationship. "Melisa, while you may not be able to see my health condition right now, except for this damned tube sticking out of my side, I hope you understand that I may get very sick. I don't know when it may happen."

"But they can fix it again, can't they? Why wouldn't you be able to get help again if it does come back?" she asked softly.

"I would hope so, but my doctors aren't making any promises, and it will have to be determined if and when it comes to that."

We left it at that. We tried to put to the side the fact that I had a chronic illness lurking. And it was sometimes easy to forget as it would subside into the background. Neither of us had any idea of what was to come, and we moved forward as best we could.

It was early 2002, and we had dated for a little over a year. We were out to dinner, and I asked her to drive by the place where we met, so I would know for sure where it was. She pulled over. It was dark and cold out.

"Melisa, I love you and want you to marry me." I had the ring and brought it out.

Now, in the movies, the prospective bride ecstatically proclaims, "YES, YES, I LOVE YOU!"

Melisa had a much more subdued reaction. I was having more

of the feeling of the theme of the Frank Sinatra song where the couple is having a delightful time... *"And then I go and spoil it all by saying something stupid like 'I love you.'"*

And in this case, I had gone way beyond that. After all of the time spent single, my excitement pushed me towards wanting to get married again. To have a younger and very healthy bride who had a good job was appealing to me. It's been said that men are like fish and are attracted to shiny things. At 41, I could be looking at sports cars, but I chose this hard-working, cute Hoosier girl.

Melisa had a lot to consider. To move my way would put her an hour away from her children's father, whom they visited regularly. But I had a plan. As she began to ask questions before responding to my proposal, I laid out my plan.

"Melisa, here's what we can do. I'll sell my house in St. Joseph, and we can buy a larger home together for our five kids in St. Joseph still. After two years, my two older daughters will graduate high school and attend college. Rachel is willing to move to Covington, Indiana, for high school. That will put us back much closer to your girl's dad. We can swing this!"

Having made my offer, we drove around Danville for a while and discussed it. I could tell she was deep in thought. I had no idea of her calculus for all the factors she had to consider. I felt that I perhaps had gotten ahead of myself. After ten years of single life, I wanted something stable. I had been honest with her and wanted her to accept me for who I was. She accepted my proposal with joy but certainly tempered with a touch of anxiety.

Melisa and I married in May of 2002, at Sidney Christian Church, Sidney, Illinois, by Reverend John Sims, our minister at the St. Joseph United Methodist Church in St. Joseph. This being our former church, they were better suited for this event, as we had the wedding and a basic cake and punch reception in the church basement. I felt happy and very in love with Melisa and her girls. Having these younger children felt very natural to me. We purchased a larger, older, bi-level home near the grade school to accommodate our family. Her mom, Sharon, and stepdad Darrell built a wall to create another bedroom and helped fix things up around the place. We had our home set up.

Just a month later, Melisa and I retreated to our bedroom as she wanted to talk. "Doug, this was a mistake. It is so much harder for my kids to visit their dad. I don't agree with how you handle your daughters. You are way more lenient than I would be."

I replied, "I agree that blending the families is much harder than I thought it would be. You have to understand that the parent-child relationship is way different when the kids are older. There is more negotiation."

After saying my spiel, I thought it over and realized that we were swimming in troubled waters. But a *mistake*? We had barely adjusted to our new living arrangement. I had learned that if your wife says there is a problem, you had better listen.

The truth of it was that our marriage didn't make life better for anyone, and it had the effect of complicating life for all parties. My kids and I had been running our own show since their mother's departure many years ago.

Melisa continued to complain. "Doug, can't you see how hard this is for me? I'm working full time, doing laundry for you and five kids, cooking, cleaning, and it's much harder for me to get the kids to their dad's for visits. I don't like this town. They were rude to me at the bank, and I couldn't find good meat at the store!"

I was immersed in complaints, and after about eight months, I started to think she was right. This was a mistake. But my feelings for her hadn't changed, and we celebrated my birthday in February 2003. I thought things might get better. Then March came, and I got sick. Very sick.

"What's wrong?" Melisa asked.

"I don't know for sure, but I feel so cold and can't get warm."

Piled with blankets, she took my temperature: 103 degrees. We were off to the ER. An old foe named primary sclerosing cholangitis came back with a vengeance. Melisa was now confronted with the terrors of me entering end-stage liver failure, as this fever episode really set me back. Treated with antibiotics and fluids, I remained in the hospital for three days. Melisa was noticeably shaken. For my daughters and I, it was an event that we had become accustomed to both pre- and post-transplant. It was part of living with a chronic disease.

A few weeks after getting out of the hospital, Melisa wanted to talk. "Doug, we made a mistake. This isn't working out. We will be leaving and moving back to Indiana. But I have a request. Can we stay here for the rest of the school year for the girls to finish out?"

I replied, "Yes, you can stay as long as you need to." I knew better than to grovel. Melisa had thought this out for some time. Sure, my sickness didn't help. But no part of this ambitious plan worked out the way we hoped. I had to try and let go while still holding out hope that she would change her mind. They left after the school year ended, and we shared a lawyer and divorced quickly and quietly.

And that chapter of life closed. She was gone. I tried to accept it. What other choice did I have?

With the fog of my distress, I made a foolish mistake. Acting on a rumor, I made an ill-informed accusation against a co-worker of Melisa's. In a cowardly move, I shared the information without investigating further or talking to the other party directly. By doing so, it didn't take long for me to receive a scathing phone call.

It was a gray, cloudy day, and my co-worker Mark Gortner and I were running a gas service to the new Public Safety Building in Monticello, Illinois. We were taking a lunch break in our large, white crew truck when my phone rang, and I rolled out of the truck.

"Swinford, did you accuse me of being involved with Melisa?" The anger was evident as he shouted into the phone. "You have caused all kinds of turmoil in my family. What a chicken-shit move to not call me and ask like a man before you told others." Before I could answer, he continued, "I can clear up who is now with her." It did involve her work, but I had the wrong party.

Shocked and surprised at the news, I apologized profusely for my mistake. I felt so dumb. I mumbled my lame excuse of having been told he was involved, but I didn't vet it out, despite knowing many people who could verify. It was almost like I didn't want to know for sure.

I climbed back in the truck. Mark looked my way. "What the hell happened? You look like you saw a ghost." I relayed a short version of what happened, and Mark started laughing. "What a dumb-ass move!" He laughed so hard that tears formed at the corner of his eyes. "Dammit, Doug, why would you do that?"

"I know, I just screwed up." Mark's laughter was infectious, and the absurdity of it kicked in. We laughed about it the rest of the day. I had remorse for the offended party, and the laugh was on me.

Indeed, that was the end of that drama. Or so I thought. A final salvo came a few days later with a phone call from a woman I will call Kathy. "Doug, my name is Kathy, and I'd like to come visit you and talk about your ex-wife Melisa."

Kathy implied the issue had to do with Melisa and her estranged husband.

"Well, Kathy, what Melisa does now is her business, but I'd be happy to talk with you."

Of course, my curiosity was piqued. A wiser and stronger spiritual man would have declined, but I wasn't above gossip or sharing someone else's misery.

When she arrived, I let her direct our visit, and we found our way to the bed that Melisa and I had shared. We sat up and talked, fully clothed.

"Doug, can you tell me what is so special about Melisa that my soon-to-be ex-husband would go for her? Is she anything special in bed? Does she give good blow jobs?"

Whoa, whoa, whoa. I expected a more general discussion about this woman's pain and disappointment. She was looking for answers and any information she could gather about my ex. I gave her R-rated answers and maybe not the X-rated ones she was looking for. The questions were so personal.

She asked how Melisa liked to be touched.

"Would you like me to show you?" I offered.

She quickly declined.

Was I really that depraved to try and exploit her in her anguish? But hey, I am a guy! Don't come into my bedroom and start talking about sex. I'm going to test the limits of your curiosity. Still, her pained expression did not indicate her desire for anything other than answers.

There is a book written about divorce called *Crazy Time*, and indeed it can be a *crazy time*. It was crazy for us even to have this conversation. Choices had been made, and they say people vote with their feet.

I empathized with her. It was hard to accept that in one of *the elections* of life, Kathy and I both lost.

I'll give Kathy credit for her tenacity. She wasn't going down without a fight, and if there were anything she could do to get her man back, she would do it.

Okay, so I failed at marriage a second time. But I tried. I was living full go. I felt compelled to push and move on.

A few months after our split, I wanted to buy a new car. I loved sports cars and had a fast V-8, four-speed on the floor Ford Mustang in my youth. And I was a single man again—mid-life crisis candidate.

Despite that, I went practical instead and came home with a new Dodge Caravan. I still had kids and their friends to haul around, after all.

Previously, Melisa urged me to get rid of the mini-van I had when we were married because it was getting old. With my new freedom, I set that straight. The hot rod could wait for a few more years. Would a sportier car enhance my position with the ladies? Either way, why bother? I had attracted plenty of trouble with my boring vans.

My oldest daughter Ashley was off to college, and Jessica became Queen Bee of the house. She and Melisa clashed somewhat when we all shared a home. Melisa saw a very bleak future for Jessi and her extroverted and strong-willed personality. Jessica's teachers and school resource officer thought she was doing great when Melisa and I visited the school to check on Jessica's progress. After Melisa left, the household calmed down, and I literally had some peace because with the kids growing up and being away at their school activities and jobs, I actually had a quiet house from time to time.

In reflection, I also felt some vindication of my concern going way back to dating Penny of how difficult it would be for any woman to fit into our complex family and health situation. My girls grew up with the variables of my illness. They had long dealt with adversity and the gaps a single father couldn't always fill. Their mom was in close touch, but it wasn't the same as living with us.

In late 2003, my health team at Barnes-Jewish decided to schedule a meeting. My big buddy Kevin "Chip" Grice and I headed down to St. Louis on the three-hour drive to figure out thc plans.

We met with my transplant coordinator. She came right to the point. "Doug, your disease has advanced, and we want to discuss the options we see for you. First off, we are confident that you can live another six months without any intervention. However, if you try for a second transplant, your rate of surviving the surgery is 50/50. It is a most complicated situation for our surgeons to do a liver transplant. With your scar tissue and general health decline, it would be high risk for you to seek another transplant."

My friend Kevin sat patiently and listened for a minute. Kevin had been a heavyweight wrestler in high school and was still a big and strong guy. He shifted in his seat. Knowing him to speak his mind, I could tell he was agitated. He belted out in an incredulous tone, "Are you telling us that you expect Doug to tell you he is going to accept playing it safe and living out six months instead of trying to get another transplant?" Kevin was obviously steamed now. I knew there was a reason I brought him.

She replied, "You have to understand that we have to explain the risks and show you the options."

I tried to answer, but she wouldn't allow it.

"No need to answer now. Call us back in about a week with your decision."

My choice was obvious. After informing the team that I wanted to go forward with a transplant, they set me up for a procedure to lower the risk of having a life-threatening bleed. I had the surgery to do the TIPS (transjugular intrahepatic portosystemic shunt) procedure to lower the blood pressure on the enlarged veins in my stomach and esophagus. The ravages of end-stage liver failure were coming home again. I was unaware of other effects that the TIPS procedure might have on my system, but I was to find out soon enough.

A few weeks after TIPS, I struggled to get up for work. I called

Bob Cain, the scheduling foreman, and said I would be late. I just couldn't wake up all the way. At around 10:00 a.m., I called Bob again and let him know I would not be in at all. I went back into a deep sleep. Rachel had cheer practice after school and was going to a friend's house after practice, and Jessica had to work at her grocery store job.

After school, Jessi came home, changed clothes, and came up to see how I was and say bye.

"Hey, Dad, are you okay?"

I didn't respond.

"Dad, I didn't know you weren't going to work today. What's wrong?" She became concerned and pressed the issue.

I could hear her but had trouble responding.

"Dad, wake up! Do you need help? Should I call an ambulance?"

I was finally able to answer. "Yes, get help. I can't get awake."

The St. Joseph-Stanton Fire Department arrived first, and for some reason, I saw these helpers as invaders and kidnappers even. I started to fight. My motor skills were so poor that I couldn't land any punches, but I was out of control and combative. Neither Jessica nor I recognized that I was going into a coma due to hepatic encephalopathy. The alarming swelling in my brain had turned me into a swearing, swinging, out-of-control, sick person. After exhausting other options, they finally restrained me and secured me with duct tape.

I yelled at my daughter. "Jessica, why did you call these people here? They are taking me to prison, and I didn't do anything!"

As the snowflakes flew outside, the paramedics tried to get me on a stretcher.

I refused at first, but eventually allowed them to take me out on one of the kitchen chairs to which they had to secure me. The firefighters were extremely kind and understanding in handling me and passed me on to the ambulance workers. Jessica surely felt upset at the scolding, but she had likely saved my life by waking me up and ensuring I was okay—I was not.

Dr. Greenberg entered my hospital room the next day. My parents stayed there with me, clearly realizing the seriousness of the situation. I lay restrained to the bed with minimal movement allowed for my arms.

Dr. Greenberg kept his distance but asked, "How are you feeling?"

My reply was swift and crisp. "I'm angry. I have been mistreated here."

"Well, now, Doug, you haven't been yourself with this mental confusion, but you seem to be clearing up. I can get the restraints off if you will cooperate," Dr. Greenberg said.

I felt better having my long-time doctor there. He always knew what to do.

I had never experienced mental confusion and paranoia like this. Even after the restraints were removed, I felt mistreated. I wanted to leave the hospital, but the staff insisted I needed to clear up my thinking and recover from this serious episode.

In response, I called my co-worker Mark Gortner, who had been with me at the jail job site when I got my tongue-lashing for spreading rumors. I looked around at the staff, including the male nurses, and I deduced that none of them could stop Mark. Mark was strong and could also deliver an attitude that would not require any physical force. So I called him and asked for help.

He suggested he would help me file a complaint after I was released instead of my strong-arm approach to get out by force. Once I was thinking straight, Mark and I could joke about all that. But at the time, I was serious.

This incident shook me. But I had already done all the testing to qualify for another transplant, and this incident put me at a higher mortality rate, which raised my MELD (Model for End-Stage Liver Disease) score higher. This all meant getting a call sooner.

A few weeks later, I was having dinner at my parents. My mom had made turkey gumbo, one of my favorites. Dad and I were reminiscing about old tales of fish both caught and lost and laughing over our various boating and camping mishaps. "Dad, do you recall we were out fishing at Marshall Lake in a jon boat, and you were trying to start that clunky little seven horsepower, and it sputtered and fell off the back of the boat?"

Dad replied with a laugh, "How can I forget? Because then I was crazy enough to jump in the lake to try and find the motor!"

That story never got old, and I can still picture it to this day. I would have loved to hear Dad explain to our neighbor Bud Severns that the motor he had loaned out lay on the bottom of Marshall Lake in about 20′ of water.

We then turned to a more serious discussion. "I talked to work, and they understand I can't come back until I get fixed up. I'm on sick leave and will file for disability. Some good news, though, my long-time friend and co-worker Veda Cooling told me last week that our church, St. Joseph United Methodist, is doing a fundraiser for us. They are doing a pork chop drive-through sale at the church. It is so kind and generous. Veda has assured me that Dottie Mercer and the prayer warriors there are praying for me too."

Mom said, "That is so nice of them to do that. That involves so much work!"

"I know, Mom. I can't express enough thanks for all that is being done for me. Wilbur Clark at work called me and said he had approval from the superintendent to raffle off another hog for us like they did in 1991. Wilbur seemed very disappointed when I declined. I knew the church had a plan, and I just didn't feel right asking my co-workers again, and besides, we aren't in quite as dire straits financially as we were in 1991."

I felt terrible for what my parents had to go through with me. In the last year, I had come to them with the sad news that Melisa and the girls would be leaving, and then they watched me descend health-wise again to where I needed another miracle. After our dinner and chat, I lay on the couch for a nap.

I woke up to my cell phone ringing. My new transplant coordinator, Pam Thurston, spoke on the other end. "Hi, Doug. We have a potential donor for you. We would like you to head on down this evening."

I called home and told Jessica that it was go time.

"Can Rachel and I go along, Dad?"

"Sure, you two are my helpers and support."

I said my goodbyes to my excited parents and collected the girls, and we were off. Ashley was away at college, but we let her know what was happening.

My daughters and I were close because of our trials over the years and a somewhat unconventional upbringing. Fate kept giving us challenges that made us grow to try and meet them.

Traffic on the street seemed light as we jumped onto I-57 South at Pesotum, and we made good time to the massive Barnes-Jewish Hospital complex in St. Louis.

The staff prepped me up, and the kids were still awake in my room with me. Both Jessi and Rachel showed interest in future medical careers and watched the professionals who attended to me very closely.

A doctor came in at 3:00 a.m. "Mr. Swinford, we are sorry to tell you that there was a problem with the donor liver, and it is a no-go. You can go back home, and we will call when we get another donor."

It was as simple as that. The kids kept their game faces. There were no tears, just resolve. The staff took out my IV, I got dressed, and we headed home.

I woke up as we rolled into the garage of our home. The girls asked almost simultaneously, "Dad, do we have to go to school today?"

"No way, let's get some rest." I managed a shower and went right to bed.

The girls and I were fast asleep after getting rebuffed in our efforts to obtain a life extension for me. The team informed me that an "offer" or call always depends on the donor organ passing tests to ensure a healthy gift.

As we slept into the afternoon on the bright sunny day, the nearby grade school emptied, and children were walking by the light traffic of the side street in front of our home. I woke and looked out as the tail end of the kids went by, chatting and joking with each other. The playfulness and innocence of the children warmed my heart. I lay back down to catch a little more rest.

The bluegrass song "O Death" would be fitting for anyone in my situation.

Well I am death, none can excel
I'll open the door to heaven or hell
Whoa, death someone would pray
Could you wait to call me another day

Yes, I could plead for another day, but this required a visit of death elsewhere. All of that was beyond my control, and I wished no one harm.

On April 13, while I dined at my parents' and before heading to the hospital, a tragedy unfolded in a suburb of the great city of St. Louis. A 59-year-old man named Bob Schwyhart arrived home from his job as a machinist. As told by his daughter Kim, his wife Jeanette called home at about 4:30 p.m. "Hey, Pa, I have a few errands to run. What are you doing?"

Bob responded in kind with the names they usually called each other. "Well, Ma, I'm folding laundry, but I don't feel good. I have a terrible headache."

"Okay, why don't you take something? I'll be home before too long," said Jeanette. After arriving home, she called her daughter Kim. "Something is wrong with your dad. It's almost like he drank too much, but I know he wasn't drinking. He didn't feel good."

"I'm coming right over, Mom."

When Kim reached her parents' home, an ambulance had already arrived, and Bob was on the stretcher but no longer talking. Kim was terrified. She had never seen her dad so sick, and he didn't have any health history to indicate what was going on.

At the hospital, the family gathered quickly and was escorted to a family room. "Bob has had a severe aneurysm, and we have lost him. He's on life support, but there is nothing we can do can restore him."

A short time later, a well-dressed woman came in to talk with them about considering organ donation. She left the room after delivering her message and allowed them privacy to decide.

Kim explained, "We all talked about how Dad liked to help people, and we decided quickly to go forward with it."

For Bob, the lyrics of "O Death" spoke as he lay on life support:

I'll close your eyes so you can't see
This very hour, come and go with me
I'm death, I come to take the soul
Leave the body and leave it cold

There was nothing fair about what happened to Bob. Was it destiny? Did Bob's appointed time to die come? Bob remained sustained on life support into the morning of April 14, while Kim and Jeanette kept a vigil with him. He was treated with the greatest dignity and moved to the transplant center. By the late afternoon, calls were going out to those in need. It just so happened that Bob and I had the same blood type and approximate body size.

My phone rang at about 3:00 p.m. I still felt a little foggy from the late night before and from sleeping much of the day. On the line, I heard Pam Thurston from the transplant office. "Doug, I'm going to ask you to come back again tonight. We have a liver for you."

I didn't know at the time, but Bob's tragedy had given me hope to see my younger two daughters graduate high school, maybe make it to their weddings, and maybe even experience the arrival of grandchildren. A whole new realm of possibilities for my life opened up because Kim and her family said, "Yes." I had a chance. In my condition, no guarantees of tomorrow existed. I was at the mercy of events over which I had no control.

For the return trip, my sister Cheryl Luts took me to the hospital, and I met Dr. William Cavanaugh Chapman late that evening.

"Hi, Mr. Swinford. I'm Dr. Chapman. I think this will work out well for you. We will get you in for surgery soon!" The doctor spoke with enthusiasm despite appearing to have been working long hours. He wore a white surgical coat, and from the stains, it was evident he had just come from surgery. His eyes were tired, and he needed a shave, but the field he was in required him to work when the planets lined up.

I felt more confident after talking with Dr. Chapman. At the time, I had no idea the impact and involvement Dr. Chapman would have on my future. I needed an extra-complicated surgery, and I had to have faith that the team would be up to the task. It was still on my mind what my previous coordinator had told me. It was a 50/50 proposition to get through surgery safely. My new coordinator Pam and my surgeon Dr. Chapman both seemed supremely confident.

In the low points of the last few months, I had accepted that I was most likely going to die. I had made all the possible arrangements for my girls that I could. My greatest concern was for my youngest daughter, Rachel. At 14, she was sensitive, and I felt she needed me. Ashley and Jessi were well on their way to independence. After the next 48 hours, we would know a lot more about what would happen.

I woke up on the evening of April 15 with my taxes paid and a new liver sewn into my body. On April 24, Dr. Chapman came into my hospital room and said, "Doug, we are pleased with your progress. You are recovering rapidly, and we are going to send you home."

I was in awe. I braced for the worst, but the delicate operation had better results than my first transplant. Techniques and immune suppression had improved significantly since 1991. There was no bypass from the upper arm to the groin to be a source of pain. I was getting around well and went home and resumed life.

It was like starting life over in a way. Before the second transplant, I conceded and accepted my fate. I had done my best. My disease came back with a vengeance. I said my prayers and preplanned my funeral. I felt the presence of my father's mother, Ruby, a Pentecostal prayer warrior and woman of faith whom I had never met because she passed some years before my birth. Such was her faith that the knowledge of it came to be passed down. My dad felt over-churched as a boy, but his love and admiration for his mother was something he shared freely. As it turned out, I skipped the trip to the morgue. Not my time yet. Dr. Chapman and the team saw to it.

I was now 44 years old and given another chance at life. I had qualified for Social Security Disability again and sick leave from my job so I could pay the bills and do what I needed to recover. This was essential because I wasn't stressing over financial matters or pushing myself too hard. My job was to get healthy and stronger and see if I could again return to physical work. And with my two older daughters almost out of the house, what was I going to do with my life? I wondered what was in store for the next chapter, as it now appeared that by the grace of God, I was able to keep living.

CHAPTER 7
LET'S CELEBRATE!

Kevin, who came along for the "talk" at Barnes with my transplant coordinator, still fumed whenever we reminisced about the subject. With the second transplant now behind me, he invited me to his house. We sat in Kevin's garage with the door open, looking out at the bursting colors of spring. He had a three-bedroom brick home in a rural area about five miles south of St. Joseph. His parents built the place in 1972, and he had made few changes since. Woods sheltered the property on the north side, and to the south, across from the house, lay a cornfield with the evidence of the recently planted corn prying through the soil to absorb the sun's rays. It made for a relaxing, bucolic background to view as we got set up to talk and usually laugh, so I could find out what was on his mind.

As it customarily did, the rustic garage smelled like a dive bar with the odor of beer and faint cigarette smoke. A Billy Bass singing fish hung on the wall, as did an outdated bikini calendar. His Blue Heeler dog Lacey came in and laid down near his feet. He was drinking Mountain Dew. Kevin was a country boy, and soft country music played in the background. In the past, horses roamed the large front part of the property. After his wife Cheryl left, he gradually lost interest in the horses. Kevin had custody of his now fifteen-year-old son, Jesse. Being we were both single parents from the time Jesse and my youngest daughter Rachel started kindergarten, he became an important confidante in all areas of life. We often talked on the phone at night after the kids went to bed. The garage offered the chance to smoke if he felt inclined, as he didn't like smoking in the house.

He stated, "Dude, I know you are down a little over all that has happened in the last couple of years. You have it made now. Melisa was a go-getter and cute, but she was kind of fussy. Putting your kids together and her having to move from her home area really complicated life for both of you. I know it hurts, but you can get another girlfriend in a half hour" (Kevin loved exaggeration.) "But I think you should just hang loose and have fun. Learn to be happy being single for, say, six months or a year. Get a hobby or hot rod car, or get a Jeep or a sports car, or something fun to shake up life. You have made a lot of progress in raising your kids these last 13 years since our old ladies split."

"I think you are right, Kevin. Lay off the dating for a while and figure out what my 'thing' is. My whole identity has become my kids and their activities, and I need to figure out where I'm going. Kevin, I just don't feel the same about some things. I don't think I've lost my faith in God, but I've kind of lost faith in people. It was only my faith in God and my desire to continue to be a dad that stood between me and death. I was idealistic in getting married young and just assumed life would work out like it did for my parents."

Kevin stopped me. "Doug, we were all young and naïve when we married. And yes, when it all goes to hell, you have to adjust your whole life to a new reality." Kevin lit a cigarette. "I think a lot of what we learned in Ralph's divorce class helped us." Kevin took a phone call from one of his many friends, and we took a little break.

As he chatted with his caller, I contemplated what I had used as coping mechanisms. Before my first transplant, I had used Bible scripture like, "I can do all things through Christ which strengthens me" (Philippians 4:13 NIV).

I recalled saying that in my mind over and over while I was at work. I couldn't think gloomy thoughts at the same time. To help stem the anxiety, I also found relief in Dr. Norman Vincent Peale and his teachings in his book *The Power of Positive Thinking.* He emphasized scriptures such as, "I have come that they might have life, and life more abundant," (John 10:10 NIV). I often recited these scriptures in my mind. I tried to dig in spiritually after Dr. Greenberg told me what we were up against 20 years prior.

Additional means of coping came through the divorce class Kevin had just mentioned. I recalled a book from our reading list by Scott Peck called *The Road Less Traveled.* The main theme I took from it was that *life is difficult, and the sooner we accept this we can deal with life more effectively.* Okay, so we should *expect* life to suck a little or a lot? But it did make sense to me. And to add to my arsenal, I read a book for a college sociology course titled *Man's Search for Meaning* by Viktor Frankl. Now there was a guy who drew a nasty lot in life. Most of his family was killed by the Nazis, and he found himself in a concentration camp with little chance of dodging the gas chamber. He faced great danger even right before the Allies liberated the camp. He later developed logotherapy, which ascribes that finding meaning in life is essential. What was most helpful to me was the idea of *what is life asking of you*? To Frankl, he had to plod along in the mud of a forced labor camp, getting barely enough to eat and regularly beaten with little chance to survive. Life was asking a high price indeed.

When I thought of the plight of those in the death camps and the soldiers who hit the beach at Normandy with a slim chance of surviving to help make the liberation possible, my psychological chafe seemed pathetic. As Kevin got off the phone, I was jostled back to the present.

I took no offense that Kevin had taken a call. Many friends called him for help, and I'm sure their need was greater at that time than his trying to pep me up.

Almost as if he was reading my thoughts, Kevin resumed the conversation. "Look, buddy roe," he loved to call friends this, "your divorce after just a year happens to people all the time. Nobody cares. I know you feel that it is a spiritual failure of sorts, and my idea of faith is different from yours. I know when I've done wrong, but I'm not into organized religion. But you sure as hell should be thanking your higher power that you are still here." He paused and took a drink of his Dew. "You need to get over yourself a little bit. Yes, you have had your hard knocks, but you are here now and in pretty damned good shape. You have good kids and a super good job. If you could drink, we would get drunk just to celebrate how freaking lucky you are!"

Few friends could be so blunt. And he was right. I needed to stop moping around. "Damn, this is a tough crowd out here. Your dog is the only one who seemed happy to see me. Are you sure you got it all off your chest?" I said with a laugh.

Kevin had laid it out. And now, it was up to me what I was going to make of the life that I now had.

Lifelong friends were not easy to come by, and I was lucky to have two greats. Kevin, Dan, and I had all known each other in high school, got married in our early twenties, and went through a divorce about the same time. Dan and I leaned on our big buddy for advice and chastisement as needed, as he had just done for me about getting over my melancholy.

Kevin was quick to call out hypocrisy as it related to Dan and me trying to maintain contact with our respective churches in the post-divorce phase. He was especially hard on Dan, who had a lot of capital with the ladies. Handsome, well-built, and charming, I felt Kevin was a bit jealous of Dan. To be fair, I probably was too.

"Hey Dan, when you took your young girlfriend to church, did anyone question if she was a friend of your daughter?"

Or, in my case, "Hey Doug, did you mention at church that you and your girlfriend were going to Las Vegas?"

Dan and I tried to be discrete about our weaknesses, but the three of us went to a strip club in one instance. Kevin didn't chide us directly but made sure to let everyone know about it. Including in front of my kids. I tried to imply that my purpose in going to such establishments was only as a "designated driver."

My older two daughters would say, "Yeah, right, Dad," with a shoulder shrug.

But Rachel took a serious tone, "Dad, you don't have any business going to bars or nightclubs. And I saw that box *of Black and Mild* little cigars in the van!" Who needed a wife with this kind of oversight? I couldn't even puff on a cigar once or twice a year!

Kevin and I talked on the phone a few weeks after our talk in his garage. "Kevin, I know I may not set the best example with some of my conduct."

Kevin responded, "Dude, don't worry about it. We are all mature adults. I respect your church stuff. I'm all good with you guys. I just like to call you and Dan out for the sake of it!"

My response to my coaching from Kevin about needing a

hobby or a fast car did not lead me to park a Ferrari or a monster truck in my driveway. I was satisfied riding around in my friends' cool stuff. Dan had a military H-1 Hummer and a Corvette, not to mention Kevin's potpourri of fun that included a Chevy four-door dually truck, a Jeep, and a four-wheel ATV. My step out of my comfort zone consisted of an on/off-road motorcycle, but it didn't have the excitement of when I had one as a youth. The kids didn't take much interest in the bike, and one of my co-workers, Ron Frye, saw me riding to work on the smoky two-stroke bike.

Ron said in a chiding voice, "So you looked death in the eye and came through, and now you are riding a mosquito-fogging death trap?"

Just missing a varmint at 50 miles an hour and getting the apprehension of distracted drivers led me to part ways with the bike. I didn't need any self-inflicted collywobbles resulting in a body all torn up.

Way more important than any fun wheels was how the three of us supported each other greatly. Wives and girlfriends came and went, but we were there for each other. My friend David had helped me out of the gate during my first transplant and marital sorrow, and we remained close, but he married Linda and moved away. Kevin, Dan, and I were most fortunate to have these enduring friendships to help us through the inevitable rough patches of life and dealing with exes.

After Kevin's garage talk and my own realization of the unique opportunities that still lay before me, I became encouraged by where I was in life. Looking for a direction, I called friend Linda Oldham about what was going on in the local dance scene since I had been absent for a few years. She was hosting dances at the downtown Champaign bar, Cowboy Monkey. She played the music, and I became interested in a dance called "West Coast Swing." Her dances were great fun and reignited my passion for dancing again. Wanting formal training, I discussed it with Dan.

"Dan, I'm thinking about going back to the Regent Ballroom to get some exercise and learn a new dance."

Dan replied enthusiastically, "Let me know how that goes because I would like to get back there to refresh some dance moves too. It is a great mix of married and single people. You should jump right in and have no trouble finding a dance partner because I think there are usually more women than men. A lot of nice people, and many are from the university. Let me know how it goes!"

CHAPTER 8

DON'T FORGET TO DANCE

I returned to the classy Regent Ballroom, located in Savoy, Illinois. I really had no idea of the wide-ranging effect that this choice would have on my life. I had taken dance lessons there in the past, and it was a delightful environment and an extremely well-managed business. David Lin and his wife Ellen hosted dance lessons, a weekly Friday night dance, and wedding parties. They also led trips and cruises to exotic places. Proper etiquette was both instructed and expected from dance participants. It was somewhat formal with a dress code for the dances, with slacks preferred over jeans. And no smoking was allowed even before Illinois law banned such activity. There was a full bar, but again, expectations were to maintain proper conduct. I had met friendly people at prior times, and Cupid did match a few couples from the ecosystem of the lessons, dances, and other activities.

In my return, I took a dance class to review the ballroom staples of swing, waltz, and foxtrot. I had my transplant in April, and this was the fall session in 2004. I was still recovering, but the dancing was good for motor skills and general exercise. It was challenging but fun to learn. It was a compelling crowd due to our diverse population, with the University of Illinois drawing students from various cultures and places. There was a mix of single and married people. It was my first chance to dance with and gain acquaintance with women from around the world, which I found most intriguing. The Regent dances were engaging settings where I could sit and talk with people and make new friends.

Reflecting on where I was, I felt my life was at a turning point. I was eager for new experiences, new travels, and to meet new people. I resumed classes at Parkland College in my long pursuit of an associate degree through night classes. In 2005, the Ballroom offered a cruise down the California coast and into ports of call in Cabo San Lucas and Puerto Vallarta. I asked my youngest daughter, Rachel, "Do you want to go on this cruise to Mexico with me? We will fly to Los Angeles and cruise to Mexico."

"Are there any kids going?" Rachel, now 15 years old, asked.

"Yes, for one, David and Ellen Lin, the trip hosts, are bringing their youngest son and daughter. I will try and book us a whale-watching trip in Cabo, and we can go into Puerto Vallarta."

"Sure, Dad, that sounds great!" I knew it was special for a dad and daughter to have this chance to travel jointly. It offered a window in time when we *could* do something like this. Given my rocky last couple of years, I was thinking more of the memories we could make than worrying about building my retirement account. The illness and hospital bed were quite educational, as they related to life's fragility and the need to capitalize on opportunities when they came. It was presumptuous even to think I would make it to retirement. And if I was favored enough, my company had a pension plan besides what I might save in a 401K. The caveat was that I had to live long enough to realize that particular benefit. There was no putting off travels to an ensuing time that I may or may not reach. Life had put the spurs to me to get with it and go see and do.

Rachel and I embarked on the beautiful Princess Cruise ship with our group of 30 on a sunny Los Angeles afternoon. It was the first time Rachel and I had ever been on a cruise ship, and we were amazed at the lavish food spreads. We were only asked about our status once. While we were in line at the food buffet, an elderly woman asked, "Are you two on your honeymoon?"

"No, ma'am, this is actually my daughter."

Rachel, who was 15, laughed and later commented, "I'm not sure how well that lady can see!"

Upon arrival in Cabo, I asked Rachel, "Are you still up for whale watching? I saw the rafts that we are going in, and they don't amount to much in relation to the size of a whale."

"Sure, Dad, I know how to swim!"

With our life jackets firmly secured, we took off. The beautiful blue of the Pacific welcomed us, and the captain explained, "While this is an inflatable raft, it is very durable. We also respect the whales and keep a safe distance, but we will most likely see gray or humpback whales. They are migratory and spend summers up north near British Columbia or Alaska."

We had maybe 10 or 12 people, but all of us were awed when we saw the massive and majestic whales breach the ocean's waters. I couldn't help but think what would happen if they came up right under us. Apparently, our guide knew how to keep a safe distance. We enjoyed the whale watching and all aspects of the trip together.

Two years later, the Regent Ballroom initiated talk of a Mediterranean cruise: Italy, Greece, and Turkey. I looked at it as a once-in-a-lifetime trip. When else would I be able to go to Rome? Would I ever make my own trip to the Grand Bazaar in Istanbul? Go to the grounds of the original Olympics in Greece? View the shores of the Amalfi Coast? David and Ellen knew how to plan a trip. I would not do this on my own, so I signed on. While I had a few dates here and there before this trip, this was not a trip to take a casual date. Given that I had no significant other, I went to the kids.

At that time, I floated the idea, and the consensus was that Jessica could have first choice. She was the only daughter who had not yet had an international trip. Ashley had been to England, France, and Spain with her high school Spanish class, and Rachel and I had our travels to Mexico. Jessi recalls that it was like this when I asked her, "Jessi, I thought I had a date lined up, but it fell through. Can you go?"

The only recollection of a possible date was a somewhat younger lady friend who had done a West Coast Swing class with me at the ballroom. We had friendly dates after dance class. We might hug or give an occasional quick kiss, but she stunned me one evening while we had ice cream. Again, we had discussed nothing about intimate matters, and I found her very attractive but not physically warm to me, so I saw us as friends.

Sitting in a booth at Dairy Queen, she prattled on about a man, whom I will call Marshall, that she had been seeing, "Marshall is a great fuck, but is a schmuck. You and I can be monogamous but not exclusive."

Wow! The key word for me was "monogamous." Did I hear that right? I was shocked at her comments as she was well-educated and appeared to be proper. I had rarely heard a woman kiss and tell with an evaluation like that. It was in the category of *too much information.* In my experience, women were usually more subtle about what they wanted. While I was eager to test the possible green light, it came with alarm bells. If we wade in intimate waters together on a Friday night, then on Saturday night, I might see her out with someone else, maybe even Marshall. So I would be trusting that our "pact" would hold up? It seemed shaky to me, given my insecurities. At the very least, I would initiate a more passionate kiss because it was just too much provocation for me to resist. But as I had told my daughter about the cruise, I did not have a *feasible* date to take

Jessi teased me with, "Why don't you go by yourself, Dad? You might meet some hot chick!" I considered the likelihood of a *Love Boat*-type romance to be very unlikely.

"Jessi, let me tell you something. Do you recall me chasing the bright lights and going to Las Vegas by myself in 2005? That just wasn't nearly as fun as if I had someone to share it with."

Indeed, I discovered on that trip that almost everyone had a friend or spouse with them. And after having great seats and listening to a Chicago concert at MGM, who was I going to talk to about it? My journal? I didn't have a journal. The trip was good people-watching, but I decided I didn't want to travel alone again.

"Well, Dad, I'm very interested in going to Europe, and this might be my main chance," Jessi said. "I'll go!"

Jessi was in nursing school, and she could be my health overseer. She added, "Dad, I'm not going to be a chaperone; you can still fall in love if you want!"

My kids loved to tease me about my non-existent love life. It was all in good fun, and I could give as well as take when it came to the teasing.

When I went for dance lessons, I had no idea that this would connect me with these most enthralling trips, and Jessica and I were amazed at the sights and historical places we visited. The dramatic sculpture in St. Peter's Basilica of Mary holding Jesus's lifeless body, as done by Michelangelo centuries before, brought an indescribable feeling. Even though I was not a practicing Catholic as I had been in my youth, the Basilica in Vatican City was the most profound part of the trip for me.

Strolling near the Coliseum, it occurred to me that I had absorbed a hell of a lot that went wrong in life. Regardless, I always clung to hope for a better day. I had made some good moves on the chess board to find myself here—with visits to Pompeii before leaving Italy, then on to Greece and Turkey still to come, not to mention we would be back to the cruise ship enjoying fine dining by this evening! It was back to what my friend Kevin told me about how lucky I was. I'd drink to that. The decision to seek a new community of friends at the Regent had taken me to great places.

Lest I think I was entering a golden age of life, I received a swift kick in the knickers shortly after the trip. There was a procedure that I had put off until after the trip, and it was corrective for what my doctors felt was scar tissue causing some blockage from my liver and causing fevers. I had the surgical procedure to install an access to my bile ducts similar to the drain I had before my second transplant. They told me that since this entered between the ribs, I could expect it to be quite painful for some time. The procedure was completed in St. Louis early in the week, and I had a party planned at my house for the weekend to celebrate the trip and show the video made by David Lin and talk about the great places we visited.

As the week progressed, I was really sore at the incision site on my right side, but home care had been by and said they thought I was healing okay. I called my local doctor, and they, too, reassured me. I called my coordinator, and they felt too that it would just take a few days.

My friend Rick called. "Hey, are we going to have the party after your surgery thing this week?"

I answered, "Sure, it has been planned for a while, and I'd like to see it through."

"You don't sound too good, but I'll help you out any way I can," Rick said.

And he added, "By the way, Debbie, Terry, and I made a video of *our trip* while you were away on your high roller trip!"

"I can't wait to see that. I'll see you Saturday afternoon," I said.

Rick came, and we had the grill set up. "Are you sure you can do this, Doug? You seem short of breath."

"Yes, I'll take some pain pills and sail right through."

Our guests arrived, and we had a good meal, and all anyone could talk about was seeing *Rick's video,* and only showed secondary interest in the scenic and historical sites that Jessica and I had seen.

I had to cut the real trip video short to accommodate the crowd, but several friends did comment that I didn't look well. Finally, we got to Rick's mock video. Their *cruise* involved a small jon boat on a small pond. They had peanut butter and jelly sandwiches for their fine dining. It was hilarious and way overshadowed our trip video. And that was okay. We all had a good time, and I was able to hit the high points of our trip and answer any questions my friends had.

That night, I had to sleep upright in a chair to be able to breathe. I told Jessi that I would call for a home health visit on Monday, which I did. They said a nurse would come Monday afternoon, but no one showed up. After another difficult night, I called early the next morning, and they apologized profusely and sent a nurse right out.

The nurse performed the usual checks, and my blood pressure was high. She then listened to my lungs. "Doug, please breathe deeply again, so I can hear your lung sounds," she said. "Are you short of breath?"

"Yes, very much so, and I have been all weekend."

"Well, I'm not getting any lung sounds on the right side. We need to get an X-ray. Your lung is not inflating properly." *No wonder I couldn't breathe right!*

My lung wasn't collapsed; rather, there was a pool of blood inside that kept it from being able to inflate. When the tube was installed, it created a "bleeder," which was only now discovered. When I called Barnes-Jewish about the issue, they were in disbelief until they saw the X-ray.

I heard from Pam. "Doug, we will need you to get down to

St. Louis immediately so we can correct that."

I had hurt like hell for a week, so I was eager to get this thing fixed.

When I was situated in my room at Barnes-Jewish, Dr. Jeffrey Crippin came into my room. "Doug, I'm really sorry. When we placed the tube in interventional radiology, we hit something that we didn't know was bleeding. Now we have to, more or less, try to find a place in your side for it to drain."

After painful efforts to do just that failed, a surgeon showed up in my room. "Doug, this blood has congealed and won't come out. We need to give you spinal sedation, and we will have to open you up in your upper rib cage area, and I will literally have to scoop out the semi-dried material."

Another doctor came in and discussed that my kidneys had not taken kindly to the elevated blood pressure and stress on the body. *Well, that's just great.*

I was out of work recovering for six weeks, and the slow decline of my renal function jumped from then on. This was 2007; they had already taken 16 years of immune suppression without much complaint. But this little episode started a worrisome trend.

Chapter 9
Empty Nest

In the early fall of 2007, I had just returned to work after the bleeding incident and surgery. After a few days of getting back into the routine, I woke with one of those throbbing headaches that I called "rim rattlers." I headed into the kitchen, seeking coffee and Tylenol.

"Hey, Dad, how are you doing? I see that you are rubbing your neck," Rachel said inquisitively.

"Yes, Rachel, it is a tough one, but I have to shake it off and get to work. Sometimes, they get better as the day goes on. I can't call off sick every time I feel bad. My work assignment is already made for today. I have to go."

"Okay, Dad, I'm off to school."

Rachel had started nursing school and assumed complete oversight of me as the only child still at home. As previously mentioned, I had been known to draw her ire if my conduct didn't meet her strict standards. Her lectures were always kind, loving, and almost funny, but I thought to myself, *I will be sure to warn her future husband that she is a tough case.*

That day my co-worker Mark Harms asked, "Are you feeling okay, Doug?"

"Just some usual stuff, Mark, with my meds and still dealing with the headaches and fevers."

Mark asked, "Doug, you always seem to keep a good attitude. How do you do that?"

Before I could answer, he continued, in a philosophical voice, "I guess that's just how life goes."

"Yes, Mark, and I've tried to accept the difficulties of life and also adopt the *What is life asking of me?* philosophy that I read in a book. But getting through all the misfortune and being there for my youngest daughter Rachel's high school graduation a few weeks ago made it all worthwhile." My mind went back to it.

Like my other daughters' graduations, the high school gym was crowded with parents, grandparents, and extended families. And the room felt steamy, as it always did when packed this full in May.

Despite the close conditions, I started to feel sentimental, recalling my oldest daughter Ashley's eighth-grade graduation. Ashley looked so grown up in her dress. I remembered holding her as a newborn. In what seemed a sliver of time, Ashley was a young woman. The warning sounded. *This period of child-rearing is going fast.*

Jessica, bold and independent as ever, moved on three years

before her little sister. Rachel had reached her time. This event was the culmination of all three having grown up. In the busyness of life, time had snuck by me faster than I could absorb it. As Rachel walked across the stage, I seemed to enter something like "thin places," what Irish Celtic Lore explains as locations where the *veil* between heaven and earth collapses. I was in my own world. My toddler, who hugged me so tightly in 1991 as I headed out to Barnes, was now a woman.

We had come a long way from then. I felt a great sense of accomplishment and *relief*. I discerned that the biggest mission that God had given me in life was fulfilled. And *that* was what kept my attitude positive. I was totally wrapped up in my thoughts and shuffled out after the ceremony. "Hey, Doug!" I turned to see Kim Blair, who had taught all three of my kids in middle school. She was facing the empty nest too and asking about dancing opportunities. Our chat brought me back to the present and I was ready to host our graduation party.

Rachel was following her sister Jessica into nursing school. All of my trials, though, had familiarized my kids with healthcare workers, and the younger two were eager for nursing careers.

Their mother played an essential role in helping the schooling all work out for the children. From when they were very young, she emphasized education and taught them all she could before they started school. They also had her study habits and concentration skills. Their mom and I were consistent in our emphasis on education for our kids.

I've heard people say, "My ex and I are best friends."

Why in the hell aren't you still married, then? It was strained between Debby and me, and we had grown far apart from our high school sweetheart days. Despite our differences, it has always been easy for me to acknowledge her influence that helped the kids be successful in their education.

I was a decent enough student but could aggravate some of my teachers. In an eighth-grade history class, the retired military officer turned teacher told me to stay after class. "Swinford, you can do well in life, but the problem is you can be a *wiseass* and could pay more attention and do less clowning around. I brought you some books about West Point Military Academy. Take these home and talk to your parents."

Years later, we had a job at the teacher's house in my utility career, and he came out as I was digging with a spade and shovel. We visited amiably, but I imagine he thought, "I tried to tell him!"

After Rachel's graduation and the party at our house, I had a doctor's appointment the next day with the unflappable Dr. Greenberg. I sat in the same office I had 24 years prior at 601 West Park, Urbana, Illinois. The framed poem with the inscription, "I treated him, but God cured him," was still there. No longer was I anxious to be in his office. He always had such an uncanny ability to gather a limited amount of information and draw precise conclusions.

He came in and looked over my records.

"Doug, you need to see a kidney specialist and manage your blood pressure more closely." After getting the serious details out of the way, a thought seemed to come into his head, and he became animated.

He started chuckling as he said, "By the way, Doug, have you tried to climb any more poles lately?" He was amused recounting the tale from a few years earlier when I had participated in a trial climbing school to "try out" for the line department.

I had limped in to see him about something else shortly after, and he asked what had happened.

"I tried a climbing school for prospective linemen. Turns out, I wasn't very good at it. The hooks I was supposed to stick in the pole kept what they call *cutting out*. For safety, they did provide a belt around the pole to keep me from falling on my head. The audacity of me even trying such a thing at 40 years old and the image of me sliding down a wooden pole made Dr. Greenberg's day, and he has teased me about it ever since.

"Dr. Greenberg, I did do one thing right. They told us if you start to go down, *do not* grab the pole or you will have big splinters in your arms! When I felt the hooks slip, I just prepared for the ride down and crunched into the big pile of wood chips at the bottom like a crash dummy. Fortunately, on the second day, my co-worker Bob Bell suggested we quit. He was doing well but I have always said he did it to save me from my demise!"

It was nice for us to have a light moment. He had seen me through a lot over the last 23 years. He, and his nurse, Melody Barber, acted as my air traffic controllers, guiding me where I needed to go. Now I needed a kidney doctor, and Dr. Greenberg picked up the phone and called upstairs to Dr. Attia, and the referral was done.

I entered the kidney department to see how best to manage my situation.

"Hi, Doug. Dr. Greenberg asked me to take a look," Dr. Attia said. "I was reading your record and see you had a recent surgery. These transplant meds and that extra strain from your bleed incident and surgery have beat up your kidneys pretty good. How much water are you drinking a day?"

I knew no matter how much I was drinking, he would say it was not enough.

I said, "Well, at least 3 or 4 bottles of water a day."

"Why don't you add another 12 ounces a day? You have moderate kidney disease but are doing fine. We will get your blood pressure managed." Dr. Attia took over that part of my care from then on.

The decreased kidney function showed mainly as increased fatigue and some minor swelling in my ankles when I ate high-sodium meals, like a plate of lasagna, which I loved. I caught a break at work with an opportunity to take a Systems Foreman job. This job would be planning and scheduling work and helping in the field only as needed. This job might prolong my career, as it wasn't as much physical work.

I kept up with dance lessons. There was a table reserved at the Regent Ballroom every Friday night dance that was referred to as the "Hodge Table." Chris and his late brother Steve Hodge, both excellent dancers, had a regular crew. "Hey, Chris, can I sit at your table tonight?" It was a Friday shortly after Rachel's graduation in 2007.

"Sure, Doug. Besides, I know you won't stay here that long. You always work both sides of the room," he teased.

"What are you implying, Chris? You know that there are ladies needing a dance on that side, too!"

"Oh, I know you are just looking out for them. But I'll tell the regulars, Bobbi (Steve's wife), Becky, Rooney, and Bea that they can have their regular spots."

"Please do, Chris, but I've seen you work a room as a single guy, so I'm just following your lead!"

Then came a new player. Kathy Fogerson. I think it was at Jim Gould's restaurant in Champaign, where David Lin was staging an off-site dance, that I saw Kathy for the first time. One of my friends leaned over and said quietly, "Hey, she's good-looking and so outgoing. Looks like Hodge has the inside track already."

And he was right. If I was to take a snapshot of the room that night and I saw Kathy, Chris was also in the picture. From what I knew, Kathy was new to the scene, and Chris liked what he saw.

Kathy also met and became good friends with a close friend of mine, Ruthie Lubkman. Together, these two were not just the *Velvet Hammer* that might lead an organization, but they were Velvet *jackhammers!* Need something done, and they could do it. They formed a team for the fundraiser event, Relay for Life, to raise funds for cancer. I wasn't trying to build a firewall against future wars, but I would want these two on my side if I was.

Chris and Kathy became a solid couple and bought a house. One night, as the Friday evening dance wound down, Chris said, "Hey, Doug, do you want to come over to our place? It's called the *Storm Cellar.*"

I arrived at the address he gave me, and to my surprise, the house had a downstairs sports bar! The entire room was well executed with bar with seating for four or five, two large TVs, music, and a dance floor. Their warm, homey gathering place was great for socializing. I enjoyed the dancing, but I liked meeting people and making new friends even more. I had always found people and their lives and stories compelling. Chris and Kathy's place was an extension of the Regent in a way, but it was more talk and laughter.

The dancing and mingling were fun, but we were all just friends there, so I decided to take a shot at internet dating. My oldest daughter Ashley graduated college and started working in a human resources position, and Jessi was nearing completion of nursing school. Rachel had started her nursing training. Maybe it was the right time. Anyway, I met a very nice lady, who I will call Marie, and we met for coffee at Starbucks. We chatted and had a good time. Marie was dressed impeccably and wore tasteful makeup. I invited her to a dance at Jim Gould's restaurant as David Lin continued to run a Tuesday night dance there. That was fun, and she met some of the dance gang.

After the dance, I walked her to her car and said, "Would you like to have dinner with me this weekend?"

"I'd like that, Doug."

Marie didn't know that much about me. My Match.com ad did not lead with, "I have had two liver transplants, and my kidney function is sketchy." In a previous profile, I tried to play cute when the profile question was "Name the celebrity you most resemble." I put down "Frankenstein." It seemed everyone was trying so hard and being so serious; how about a little levity? Responses stopped coming in. *Hey, I was just kidding, going for a laugh. Besides I don't look like Frankenstein. He is tall and I'm not!*

This foray into dating was a far cry from my first dating experience after the kids' mom left, where I met the gal in the lab, and she knew I was a transplant patient. How would I share that kind of news, and when?

After our dinner date, Marie and I went back to my place to watch a movie. It was warm and snuggly. That night, while taking her home, I felt it only fair to give her some information on my condition. I may have thought she was a little out of my league, and felt a connection and desire that we may be close to becoming more intimate. In the darkness, driving her home without seeing her reaction, I stated, "Marie, I had a very nice time tonight and really enjoyed our dinner and hanging out.

"Me too, Doug. I have been enjoying our time together," she said softly and rested her hand on my shoulder.

Reluctantly, I pushed on with the facts. "Marie, I just felt that I should tell you that I have a complicated health history. I have had two liver transplants due to a disease called primary sclerosing cholangitis."

It fell quiet, and I let it be so. We had a warm kiss goodnight, and I headed home, not knowing how it would come out. Was it the wrong time? Too soon? Acting like it was more serious than I should have? I didn't know what the right thing to do was. Engaging that topic *after* becoming more intimate didn't seem fair. And don't mistake the move as high morals. Dating over your head with undisclosed liabilities is a recipe for heartbreak.

Two days later, I got the break-up letter in the form of an e-mail. "Doug, I had a great time getting to know you, but I'm not going to be able to go through with the dance lessons we had planned. I have had some issues come up in my life and need to concentrate on things at home."

She remained interested in me right up to the point that I disclosed my problems. And that was okay. I had some major health "baggage." It was understandable, and while I may have found a better way or time to discuss it, let's face it, I needed just to get it out there and see where I stood.

I knew that my health condition might keep me single, but wild horses couldn't stop me from keeping an eye out for the ladies. I joined eHarmony, which went a little deeper into personality traits. I met some nice people that way too, but nothing lasting. I was doing okay. My daughter Rachel was now working the desk at the Regent Ballroom while also in nursing school. She was great at the front desk with her smiles and happy disposition. Always the fixer-upper, she kept an eye out for ladies she thought I might be interested in.

Chapter 10

"Smooth" Moves

I was at a dance lesson on a Friday night before the regular dance and came out to talk to Rachel at the front desk after the lesson. "Hey, Rotten, how is it going so far this evening?"

My late dad had affectionately given her the nickname as in *spoiled rotten*. "It's going good, Dad. How was dance class with Rosemary?"

"Ballroom 3 is good. I'm picking up some new moves and just need to practice." While talking, I spied two ladies I had not seen before sitting in the lobby, waiting to go in when it was time for the dance. The older lady was probably in her 70s. The younger of the two appeared to be about my age or a little younger. I saw that she had a black flared skirt and a pink blouse. With shoulder-length dark hair and a lovely tone to her skin, I guessed she was Hispanic or even Native American. I was interested in asking her to dance and maybe talking to her a little bit.

The dance started, and I approached her and asked, "Would you like to do a cha-cha with me?"

She seemed a bit shy but answered, "Sure."

"My name is Doug. Nice to meet you."

"My name is Lynne."

As the Santana song "Smooth" played, I counted in my head. *One, two, cha cha cha.* She had a great natural movement of her hips and body. She caught me off-guard with a question. "How old are you?"

That surprised me as being forward and certainly a question a man dare not ask a woman. She had a very sweet accent that I guessed as Asian. "Well, I'm 49 years old."

"Oh, you are young."

Okay, so she was telling me that she was older than me. Not a big deal to me. She couldn't be that much older.

As the night progressed, another gentleman took up a lot of her time and dances; and as I understood later, told her that I was married and had three kids. He was right about the three kids.

To be polite, I danced with her friend Pauline. "Pauline, I'm happy that you came tonight." As we tried to negotiate a foxtrot to Frank Sinatra singing "New York, New York," I had to go slow because Pauline wore flip-flops and had trouble going backward. "I should have worn better dancing shoes!" Pauline said.

I was quite intrigued at first glance of Lynne and even more so after our first dance. From there, I introduced her to the owner David Lin, who was playing the music in the front of the ballroom. I took her out to the lobby to meet my daughter Rachel.

"Rachel, this is Lynne."

"Hi!" Rachel said in her animated manner. "So nice to meet you, Lynne. I saw you and your friend come in. This is your first time here, isn't it?" I wanted Lynne to have a good time and come back.

We were walking back to her table after a dance, and I said, "Could I have your phone number, so we can stay in touch?"

I watched her expression in the low light of the ballroom as she pondered for a minute. "Maybe next time." English was a second language for her, but her meaning was clear to me, and I respected her boundaries.

Having had my share of rejections, I wasn't sure how to get to know Lynne, but I wasn't going to let a little apprehension get in the way. She was polite and friendly, but I wasn't sure of her interest level. I also knew full well that to try and date also would lead to the inevitable conversation about my personal albatross. My next opportunity to possibly see her was to return to the Friday night dance the following week. My daughter Rachel asked me after work on the following Friday, "Hey, Dad, will I see you at the dance tonight?"

"I would like to go, but I had a hard day at work. And I'm so tired I think I will stay home and watch a movie."

Rachel replied, "But, Dad, I thought you would try and see if that cute gal you introduced me to last week was there?"

"How about this? If she comes to the dance, why don't you

text me, and I'll try and make it up there."

Rachel smiled and said, "Sure, Dad, I can do that."

I was relaxing and my movie, *Gran Torino* with Clint Eastwood, had just finished when Rachel came bouncing in from working at the dance. I hadn't heard a thing from her, so I asked how it went.

"It was good. Jay Voyles came out, and we talked quite a bit. Remember, I dated his grandson?"

"Oh yes, that's right."

"So I'm assuming that Lynne wasn't there?"

Rachel chuckled and answered, "About that. I'm sorry, Dad. I forgot to call you, but yes, she was there."

"Rachel, you were supposed to let me know," I protested with a smile and raised my hands. "Oh well. It isn't that big of a deal. I'll surely run into her again. And I gave her a business card with my phone number and email if she really wants to connect."

I did return the following week and was out front paying and chatting with Rachel when Lynne came out from the dance floor and said, "Where have you been? You can come and sit with Pauline and me."

Okay, so she remembers me. After paying my way, I went around the corner into the separate area that was the ballroom. The large rectangular room had a smooth wooden dance floor. The floor always looked freshly buffed. Tables and chairs lined the walls, the lighting dim with a candle at each table. The bar sat right inside the room. On dance nights, the low lighting and soft music made for a romantic setting.

Lynne was out dancing already, and I took a seat, and Pauline started giving me all the details about Lynne as only an elderly person would. I had no doubt she was dealing straight with me. "Lynne is a really hard worker and saves her money. She owns and takes care of her own home. She is a good person and friend to me. She has been talking about you."

Of course, Lynne would have been mortified had she known that Pauline was talking about her and sharing so many personal details. I just let her talk.

I needed someone stable and able to deal with all manner of adversity. In talking with Lynne, I found out she was born and raised in the Philippines. "My mom was born on the Hawaiian island of Oahu in 1920, and when Hawaii became a state, she acquired U.S. citizenship. My mother's parents decided to move back to the Philippines in the 1930s, where she met my dad. Mom always wanted to go back to Hawaii and told me she planned to go when Romeo and I, the youngest of six kids, were raised up and she could save the money. My dad Viktor, born and raised in the Philippines, couldn't be persuaded to go, and I had stayed single, so I could go to Hawaii. From the way Mom's eyes would light up about the island, I knew it had to be a special place, and I wanted to go to the United States and establish my citizenship."

I found her background compelling and encouraged her to

talk more about it. "It was difficult for us to put food on the table. We lived near Iligan City but didn't have electricity until I was in high school. We had a small farm that we all worked at to provide fruit. My younger brother Romeo often skipped school and went fishing but brought home food to go with the vegetables grown in Mom's garden. We always had rice to eat. My dad worked in an ammonia factory, which seemed to lead to his health declining." Lynne's family had also been scarred by the Japanese occupation of the Philippines in World War II.

Later, after Lynne and I started dating, I discussed the war with Lynne's late brother Carlos when we visited him and his wife Sheila in their Beverly Hills, Florida, home in 2010. He recalled in his broken English, "There was fear when the Japanese destroyers appeared off the coast, and I remember my uncle being tied up. I tried to help get ants off of him. My mother knew or befriended one of the Japanese officers and our village received better treatment." Obviously, this was a traumatic experience, which came just after the Pearl Harbor attack in December 1941, and the liberation didn't start until late 1944.

Needless to say, Lynne's family had a culture of toughness born of hardship. I greatly respect her background and how it affected her life even though she was born some years after the war. She certainly was not a spoiled woman. We seemed to click that second night we saw each other at the dance. Having had time to marinate our interactions from our first meeting, she must have concluded that maybe I was up to scratch. We set up our first date, and it was two-fold. She invited me to a Filipino-American picnic, and later that evening, we attended the wedding and party of Rachel's close friend Carli Garrison. We were having fun doing things together. After a few dates, I tried to kiss her good night, and she tucked her chin down. No big deal. It would move slowly.

She had been divorced from Robert Taylor for five years but still wasn't eager to get into anything serious.

As we discussed our trials and tribulations in the first few weeks of dating, Lynne shared more about her life in Hawaii and working in food service at Puller Hall on Pearl Harbor Naval Base. Robert was in the Marine Corps and resided in the barracks on base.

I was impressed that Lynne lived with her mother in Wahiawa for ten more years after leaving the Philippines before getting married. Gliceria, her mother, had said with a slight shake of the head every now and again, "I don't know if you will ever get married!" It mattered to me that Lynne was freethinking. Her two sisters both married young, as was the custom. Lynne liked working her various jobs and saving her money. Robert was tall and *gwapo.* Lynne showed me his striking photo in his military uniform. He was younger than her by almost a decade, but they took the leap and moved to Robert's hometown of Arthur, Illinois, which also was home to a large Amish community. I can't imagine the culture shock. From the bustling cosmopolitan city of Honolulu to the throwback scenes of horse and buggy traffic moving *clip-clop* up and down Vine Street through the heart of town.

I listened intently as Lynne gave voice to her life's details. Expressing her story was peaceful and perhaps cathartic. It was like the serenity of water moving gently over a spillway.

She had spoken so freely that I didn't have any apprehension about sharing my heavy stuff, which had ended some promising dating experiences. Worse-case scenario, I felt that we would stay friends. And with that, I brought up the topic of what had transpired with my health. "Lynne, I have a rough health history and had a second liver transplant just a few years ago. I'm doing good now but don't know how long it will last."

Her questions were direct to the point, as in, "Why did this happen to you? What are the chances it will happen again? Are you feeling okay now?"

"Lynne, it is all very uncertain. I'm okay now, but this disease has brought me down twice. Most likely, it will again, and that is why I wanted to tell you. If you don't want to continue, I understand. Primary sclerosing cholangitis will most likely take my life someday. All I can do is follow my doctor's guidance and do the best with the situation that I can."

In 2008, I had discussed with my Barnes-Jewish doctor Dr. Kevin Korenblat if I might eventually need a third transplant someday. "We are doing our best to keep you healthy, Doug, but no, there won't be any third transplant."

I repeated that conversation to Lynne. "Lynne, I will do my best, but this disease process is beyond my control. The truth is no one can predict how it will play out. Possibly they will discover a better treatment. Maybe they will have advances to be able to do further transplants. I sure hope that I don't have to go through another one. I just know that I enjoy being with you and hope it can continue."

Chapter 11

Hawaiian Wedding Song

There was no *Dear John* letter, text, or ghosting me after I told her the truth. And so, we had a thing going. We both enjoyed dancing, and she was a flamboyant dancer and could dance the *hula* with moves she had learned between 20 years growing up in the Philippines and ten years living in Hawaii. I had been trained in some dance moves. She was a natural dancer and drew attention whenever we went out.

After a few months, Lynne had her first initiation into being around when my health acted up. We were getting ready to go out on a Saturday night to dance, and I started feeling cold.

"What is wrong?" Lynne felt my burning forehead. "What can I do?"

"Just get me more covers. I'm so cold."

She covered me up on the couch, but I started shaking with chills and a fever. I took my normal medications and rode it out, but most important to me was her reaction. She was calm. She took care of me as best she could. She wasn't sore that we couldn't go out, and she watched TV and checked on me. It was nice not to feel like I was on the chopping block as my health acted up. It was a reality with PSC that I just couldn't seem to escape.

I recalled another dating situation some years prior where I was watching a movie with a date, and it was an hour drive home. I came down with one of these vicious fevers, and my date, fearing I was contagious, couldn't get me out of her house quickly enough. "Doug, you need to go. I can't be sick and miss work. I'll get your coat." As I entered the apartment building hallway, my senses seemed to absorb the sound coming from other apartments. The televisions, the music, the laughter. As I stepped outdoors, already feeling the effects of the fever, the 20-degree air hit my face. I shuffled to the car and let the engine warm up until it was hot in the car. I waited until my chills allowed me to steer the car and slowly trekked home. Needless to say, this did not endear me to this woman.

Lynne was the exact opposite. She was compassionate and accepting that I had a disease that could strike me at any time and could have long-term implications. I hoped that she would never have to see end-stage liver failure. I was taking the best care that I could to prolong the life of my gift.

It took time to gain Lynne's love and trust and time for me to trust my own feelings. I loved her and could not imagine life without her. One night after about four years of dating, I handed her a heavy, wrapped gift as we sat on the couch. She tore the paper off to reveal a patio block I had decorated. "Thanks, honey. I will put this in my garden for a step." Then she saw words in the mix of tiles, shells, and colored stones and saw the, "Will you marry me?" I was watching her face and the moment she understood what the craft project was really about was priceless.

We married on the Hawaiian Island of Oahu in 2013, a beautiful affair officiated by Captain Howie at his Waimanalo wedding venue very near the beach of the Pacific. He had a fantastic setup with vendors for hair, makeup, music, and photography, including photos on the beach. As we left on our cruise of the islands a few days later, I had to pinch myself to believe all the joy we were experiencing.

I had delighted in our dating and marriage, taking her places she had not visited, like Las Vegas, The Grand Canyon, Pikes Peak, Washington DC, including the White House, Niagara Falls, and the CN Tower in Toronto. I hoped and prayed to stay with stable health, but rumblings kept coming. The concerns about kidney function continued. And just prior to our marriage came word of a cancer threat.

I took the phone call in the office at work, and it surprised me that it was Dr. Ramkumar. He had handled a recent procedure and said flatly that the results showed what was called post-transplant lymphoproliferative disease. In other words, he called it a "plasma cell cancer." I was quite shaken at the news, and he suggested I see an oncologist.

I kept the news under wraps that day and told no one until I had an appointment after work at the periodontist. She had me meet in her office to discuss what our plan was for the work she was doing. We sat down in her small office. She said, "Doug, are you okay? You seem distracted."

I just came out with, "I have cancer." I had a momentary breakdown.

She just happened to be the person in front of me when it came out, and I guess I felt more comfortable being she was a professional. I needed to talk about it a little before I could even tell my family.

"Now, Mr. Swinford, I'm sorry to hear about this diagnosis. Surely, you are aware of the great strides in treatment for all forms of cancer?"

I had been slumped defeatedly in my chair, but her encouraging words after being able to tell someone helped me feel better.

Anyone taking immune suppression is obviously at higher risk for cancer. The suppression targets some of the good guys who fight off cancer. The oncologist, Dr. Kahl, explained it like this, "Currently, your immune system is holding this in check. If I could get you off immune suppression for a month, we could probably eliminate the abnormal cells. That would likely destroy your transplant, so we can't do that. Let's keep an eye on it. This can turn into multiple myeloma."

Shortly after my diagnosis in mid-2014, I received a phone call from my friend Kevin. "Hey, Kevin. What is going on?"

Kevin's voice was shaky. I could tell something was wrong.

"I just got on my online records, and my biopsy results are in."

A long pause ensued, and I could hear his breathing was uneven. Then his quivering voice resumed, "I have liver cancer."

"I will be right there." I pulled my shoes on, jumped in the van, and headed right out. I just wanted to listen and see where to go from here. He had a really tough road ahead with a far-advanced case.

He took ill during treatment about a year later, and I went to see him in the hospital on July 22, 2015. The elevator door opened, and there stood my friend Dan who was just leaving. "Hey, I'll go back up with you to visit for a few minutes so we are all together again."

"Thanks, Dan. Let's cheer him up a little."

Dan gave a heartfelt goodbye, and Kevin and I chatted until he got tired. I went to shake Kevin's bandaged-up hand to say goodbye. At the same time, we said, "Love you".

I choked up as I left. I reflected on the March birthday party that his long-time friends Todd and Angie Albers had for him at their machine shed. He didn't feel well but so many friends attended and his tears and laughter were shared one last time. The day after my hospital visit, he passed away.

Lynne and my kids had taken my cancer diagnosis in stride. My initial frantic thought was, *First off, I survived multiple transplants, and now this damned cancer will get me. It just claimed one of my closest friends, and he was a lot tougher than me!*

The plasma cell issue was on the observation list and stayed in the background. I was more fortunate than Kevin had been, and a number of life events with kids, marriages, and grandkids took center stage for several years and brought great happiness. And despite any health concerns, or maybe because of them, I kept pushing for new experiences.

My wife had heard a bucket list item that I wanted to plan. "Honey, do you remember when I went to the Indianapolis Motor Speedway and did a ride-along in the race car?"

Before she could answer, I continued excitedly. "What I *really* wanted to do was to *drive* one of those cars."

She didn't protest at all. "Okay, where do you want to do it?"

"Well, I can't imagine a better place than the track at Daytona Beach, Florida." I was referring to the home of the top race of the NASCAR season, the Daytona 500. The high banked 2.5-mile oval was ideal for high speeds. My wife asked, as she often did when we went to a new place, "Do they have somewhere to dance? And do they have Goodwill stores there?"

We took off to Florida and stayed near the racetrack. We entered the track on a sunny morning through the tunnel. First off, I was fitted for a driver's fire suit. The group I was with entered class, and a stocky middle-aged man started our instruction. He was a gregarious fellow with a ginger tint to his hair and a freckled complexion. "Guys and gals, I'm here to talk about your driving experience. You will drive with an instructor in the passenger's seat. I used to be an instructor before the head injury."

I took that as a joke because he said it light-heartedly. We all knew the danger of the track. It had claimed one of the best NASCAR drivers ever, Dale Earnhardt Sr., in 2001.

"Now, since you are the first class today, I'm going to take a few of the drivers at a time in the crew cab and drive you around and tell you how to get around here!"

The pit area, where we accessed the cars, smelled of oil, gas, and exhaust. It was a sunny day, but the stands looked odd because there were no spectators.

"Okay, Doug, you can climb in," said our helper.

Even though I was a slim guy, these cars have no doors, and it took some effort, but I managed to slither in and get hooked up.

In my headset, the instructor said, "Okay, fire her up and throttle up to 1500 rpm and let the clutch out and turn it loose." I don't think I was half as crazy as the professional driver riding along to *coach* me. He had no steering wheel or brake but could limit my speed if needed. I didn't mention that I had been having some vision problems. No need to cause excessive worry, right?

I discovered that this was not intended to be a Sunday drive. I was to go as fast as I possibly could. It feels great to let loose 550 horsepower and absorb the roar of the engine while barreling down the long straightaway. The problem is there is a corner at the end that looks like a wall. "Gas up! Gas up! Don't let off going into the corner," my teacher exclaimed. But with a 31-degree banked corner to negotiate, I did what I always do at corners. I slowed down.

Most certainly, it was an exhilarating experience. But when my 20 miles over eight laps were complete, I was relieved that I stayed off the wall. My instructor seemed disappointed that he couldn't get me full throttle through the corners, but I was satisfied. I had my experience. While reaching speeds of 140 mph on the track, my problems couldn't be further from my mind. They allowed Lynne to be in the pits and take pictures and videos of me driving on the track.

But her real delight had been in the dancing at the *Rockin' Ranch* in Ormond Beach the night before. She fit right in with the line dancers tightly packed on the floor. The music was great, and she was in a groove. I had to drag her sweaty self aside at midnight to get some rest for the big event at the track the following day. (I should have closed the bar down because all I did was toss and turn all night, worrying about driving on the big track.)

I completed my racecar bucket list experience! Good thing because as we moved through the summer of 2018, my lab work showed ominous signs that my kidneys were getting tired.

I had to stand for an annual physical to renew my medical card for the commercial driver's license required to do my job. I waited and waited for the doctor to come in. His computer desk was right outside the door, and he spoke to the nurse in hushed tones. When he finally came in he said, "Mr. Swinford, I have been doing your physicals for several years now, and I admire your determination to keep working. But I can't pass you due to your kidney function. You need a kidney transplant," he said in a pleading way. "I know this has major implications for your job, but I'm going to have to rescind your card immediately, and I need to speak with your supervisor. Have you considered disability?"

"Doctor, I feel that I can still work. I admit I need a lot of rest, but I can still do my job overall. And I need to check with my physicians and see if I need to do the workup for a transplant. They hadn't indicated that we were in that territory."

I was chapped at the doctor. He wasn't a renal specialist. What did he know? What did he see in the monthly lab work that was so bad?

A few months later, I did exactly what he had asked. My doctors were having me worked up for a new kidney.

"Sir, we will need to attach these monitors while you pick up speed on the treadmill."

The room looked like a mini-gym but with multiple monitors. Once all wired up, I started in and immediately felt my heavy legs. I was carrying about ten extra pounds of fluid in my lower extremities.

"Okay, sir. Increase your speed more as we are testing your heart."

After a few struggling moments, the tech had me get off and lie down, and she used other monitors to look at my heart. After that, it was lung function, lab draws, and scans as needed. It was an exhaustive process.

My evaluation came in the mail, where I received a billet-doux that stated, "Dear Mr. Swinford, we regret to inform you that due to the advance of your liver disease, you do not qualify for a kidney transplant."

I told Lynne, "Honey, I'm not that surprised. I thought I had failed the treadmill test, but I guess my PSC is winning again.

"What are we going to do?" Lynne continued. "That swelling in your ankles and lower legs is getting worse."

"I know. The liver team thought I would be able to get a kidney. I'm not sure what to do next. I have always been able to find a solution before. I still feel good enough to work. I recall our former mayor B.J. Hackler quoting his wife when a tough spot was encountered. Her saying was, 'Suck it up, buttercup, and move on!'

"I guess that is where we are at, honey. I'm sorry."

Chapter 12

When the Wheels Fell Off

I first walked through the doors of Illinois Power Company in 1979 at the age of 19 years old. I was a naïve, skinny kid who had been somewhat sheltered by my small-town upbringing. Illinois Power was a great place to earn a living and broaden my horizons by serving a large international college population and an overall diverse community. A first day turned into a week, weeks into months, and then the years unfolded. I grew up working at this company. I had experienced marriages, divorces, the joy of new life, and the sadness of lost loved ones. The one constant was I always came here, no matter what else was going on, and had formed many strong bonds.

The company name changed over the years and became part of Ameren in 2005, and I hoped to reach the finish line and retire at age 62. At 58, I was certainly getting close. Not passing my physical and losing my medical card was a game changer. I left the doctor's office that day in August 2018, and all I could do was wait to see my employer's response. It didn't take long.

The next day my superintendent Bob Elliott came by my desk and said, "Do you have a minute?"

"Sure, Bob. I'll be right there."

The topic of conversation was no mystery. My little visit with the doctor cracked the shell of denial I was operating under to keep sailing on for a couple of more years. Bob and I had a history, having both been with the company for many years and working together in the field. But he was the boss now. He had a serious look on his face. "Doug, we will have to make some adjustments and work with labor relations to see how to move forward. You will have to give up the new truck and take either of the two trucks we have that you can legally drive."

"Okay, Bob. I will take the older pickup truck; it's easy to work off of." The time came to say bye-bye to the brawny new Ford F-350 4x4. The big Ford set so high that I had to stand on the front bumper just to check the oil. It was humbling, but I felt happy to be able to keep working while my status remained under evaluation. The well-worn Chevy light-duty truck worked just fine for me.

Further updates on my status stayed quiet from August into the New Year of 2019. The first week back after the holiday, Bob summoned me again. I sensed a change about to happen. I felt that Bob had sincerely done all that he could. "Doug, I can't comment specifically, but you have a meeting this morning. A conference has been called with the managers of labor relations and human resources. They traveled from their offices in St. Louis to meet with you."

My fellow workers considered that when labor relations came, something bad was going to happen. I knew that I didn't have much time, but I wanted to say quick goodbyes to some of the operations clerks. The crews had likely pulled out already, but gas trouble-man Bob "Hawk" Hawkins was still around and was talking to Andrea, one of the staff I wanted a word with. Andrea Laley's official duties were handling payroll for the electric department. She also acted as a counselor/advocate for troubled souls. About the age of my daughters, her gift was empathy with a pretty smile, but she was tough too and could be a scold if required. Hawk was a helpful friend to co-workers, but a challenging project for Andrea. He was given to hard landings in romantic relationships as well as various motor vehicle incidences, including a souped-up mini-bike with the equivalent of a V-8 engine that left him injured. I just wanted to offer a quick thanks for her listening to *my* travails. Hawk was dispatched to a leak call.

"I have a meeting."

"I heard," Andrea said.

I heard the voice of my union rep, so I turned and only got a quick, "See ya," to Makiba, Erin, and my step-daughter, Amber. I would just have to text later for anything left unspoken.

As I walked in with my I.B.E. W Local 51 union rep, Tony Cook, I understood that this might be my last day working there.

Here we go again, another consequential meeting, all because of my health. Did I hate myself for it? How could I engage in self-loathing or self-pity, for that matter? Who was to blame? Can it be anything else than one of those mysteries of life that we chalk up to, as my father referred to it, "Just one of those things?" The impact came in increments, but the disease was starting to gain little victories against life issues that were very important to me.

At first, I felt disappointed at the doctor who failed me on my physical, but since getting shut down in my quest for a kidney transplant, I came to terms with the fact that my condition was serious. If I read between the lines, the letter from the hospital meant, "Mr. Swinford, you are too sick to get a new kidney." I had pursued what the company doctor asked me to do but was shut down in that effort as well. Now back at work, I had to stand for a meeting about my fate.

"Mr. Swinford we are here today to discuss your 'options' in regard to your employment. We give all due respect that you have had a long career of steady service. However, given that you failed your medical card for your commercial driver's license, you no longer meet the fit-for-duty requirements to do your job. Your options are to retire, go on sick leave and file for disability, or bump into a lower classification."

I was at least going to raise my only argument.

"Doesn't the Americans with Disability Act apply in this case? Couldn't my duties be modified slightly so I could continue working?"

The HR woman spoke up. "No, we are not able to make exceptions for you not having a medical card."

I was aware of exceptions that had been made in the past, but I also had co-workers who lost their CDL due to various reasons, and they had been escorted off the property when they couldn't recover the license in a timely fashion. They offered me better options than that. The problem was not the rules. It was *my* failing health that made this meeting a *fait accompli.*

"Okay, I am electing to go on sick leave and file disability. I don't want to leave my department. When I have been sick before, I had to go on disability but have always been able to recover and come back to my job."

The labor relations manager explained, "Mr. Swinford, if you have a doctor that views this differently and feels you can come back safely, and you bring me a medical card, we will put you back to work. We just don't have any other options right now. You can discuss this with Tony for a few minutes and gather a few things, but you do need to leave the property now, and we will notify payroll you are sick until further notice."

Okay, there it was. My career was slipping through my fingers. But I just didn't feel done. This job was part of my identity. This is where I was expected to show up for my assignments for the last 40 years. I stopped by my desk and handed off my work packets to co-foreman Les Storm. Les and I knew that this outcome was likely, so we had planned for it. He wished me well and I walked to my car slowly, crestfallen and humbled. One of the ladies from the office came out and expressed her sincere concern, which I greatly appreciated. I was going to miss many of the people I worked with all these years. Doors were closing. Whether it was showing up to work or asking for a new kidney, the response was the same.

I still hung on to the words, "Get someone to pass you and we can put you back to work." It was as if he knew a different doctor might see it differently. After all, how did all truck drivers pass, including some that didn't look too healthy either? Maybe it was for the best; I was scheduled to have surgery to fix multiple hernias in my array of abdominal sutures. After my belly received some patching up, maybe I could see another occupational medicine doctor.

A few months later, after my hernia surgery healed, I sat in the parking lot of a doctor I selected to evaluate me for a medical card. I hesitated before going in. I was thinking how foolish to present this to another MD. It would be quite difficult for this doctor to approve me when two that the company paid had failed me. This was my last chance.

"Doctor, I'm trying hard to return to work. Among my other health concerns has been my ability to lift anything heavy with the multiple hernias. Those have been fixed. But to be straight up, I have been evaluated by two doctors in the last six months, and they have determined that I am not able to pass for a medical card due to my kidney function. I have also been turned down for a kidney transplant." I looked directly at him while explaining and shifting the burden to the doctor in the midst of my health woes and my anxieties about the series of losses I was encountering. Was there a subconscious emotional appeal? I suppose so, but it wasn't intentional, and I felt I made a decent presentation physically, with only my swollen ankles obvious evidence of my general health.

The doctor allowed me to vent but focused on my physical exam. He asked a lot of questions. He concluded with, "I have had my own share of setbacks and understand your desire to continue your career. I am willing to work with you. Your kidney function is concerning but not in the range for dialysis. I can give you a six-month card, but you will lose your eligibility if you have to go on dialysis. And you have to be honest with yourself." He raised his hands and used them to emphasize this next part. "If the fatigue and edema become too much, you must stop working. You will likely know when that point comes. There will be a point when full focus on your health is the most important thing."

Card in hand, I motored right to my office. I presented said card to my shocked supervisor, Matt Anderson. "Wow, I wasn't expecting that you would ever be able to come back!"

"Nor did I, Matt. I'm really happy to get the opportunity to try." Matt continued to look at the paper and said, "Let me call

HR, and I'll get back to you."

I went home feeling elated and told my wife I might be going back to work. Sure enough, the labor relations manager's word held. Matt called with the good news. "Doug, you can report to work tomorrow!"

I resumed working and tried coping with the fatigue for a few months, but my renal function continued to decline. I decided to see Dr. Greenberg for evaluation and advice.

Dr. Greenberg had been my overseer and gastroenterologist for 34 years. He had become iconic in his field, and the department was now the Dr. Eugene Greenberg Institute of Digestive Health. I felt privileged to be his patient. I wanted to know if he thought I should hang it up. He was now 86. Surely an advocate to continue working, right? "Dr. Greenberg, what do you think of my general health and if I should keep trying to work? My employer has mentioned retirement or disability."

He looked at the numbers on the computer as he had many years ago when first making a diagnosis. "Why *wouldn't* you take disability?" he asked. "Surely you would qualify. The immune suppression has damaged your kidneys, and you have cirrhosis due to PSC. I think it is time for you to focus full time on your health and maybe do some traveling."

"Thank you, Dr. Greenberg."

Yikes, I always hated the word "cirrhosis" since it seemed to infer being an alcoholic. I couldn't fill a Pepsi can with the amount of alcohol I had consumed in the last 30 years. But just hearing that word caused pain in the direction of the delicate organ. The multiple organ distress left me with a constant cloak of fatigue. It was a wrestling match in the morning as I could barely get my steel-toed Red Wing boots on over my grape-fruit-sized ankles.

I worked a few more weeks. In addition to my physical struggle, I worried about the effects of the disease on my cognitive function. At any minute, I could be thrust into a situation with a blowing gas main or a house full of gas and have seconds to decide what to do. The last thing I wanted to do was hurt a fellow worker or the public I was supposed to protect.

On Friday, August 9, 2019, I called my wife and asked her to pick me up. My wife picked me up after work, and when I got in the car, she said, "Won't you need your truck in case you get a callout this weekend?"

"No, I think I'm done."

"What do you mean?" she asked.

"I mean, I don't think I can work anymore."

"Okay," she said with only one minor protestation. "Hey, I just bought new work boots and shined them all up for you."

"Yes, they look great. Thanks, honey." And that was that. My co-workers put together a send-off party at work a few months later, right before COVID-19 broke out worldwide. We also had a little after-party at a local restaurant. My co-workers had been wonderfully supportive and gave us a most generous going-away cash gift. We felt stunned and so appreciative and knew no matter what was to come, they were behind us.

I found myself in new territory. I bounced back after my transplant surgeries in 1991 and 2004. In cheating death a little by getting substitute organs, we had to compromise the kidneys with the strong immune suppression meds. The FK-506, now called Prograf, had not had me howling at the moon in werewolf mode as the nurse had joked 28 years prior. Along with the kidney trouble, my vision evolved into a moderate impairment. I underwent one successful and one failed cataract surgery, and macular degeneration was added to my list of diagnoses. With the reality of my situation, I accepted there would not likely be any comeback this time. It was time to rescue whatever potential life I had left.

My kidney doctor mentioned getting a graft or fistula to place dialysis needles for the therapy in July 2019, and brought it up several other times. In December, four months after I had left work, my artificial graft was placed at Barnes-Jewish Hospital. The surgeons put an artificial vein in my upper left arm and hooked it up to my blood system. A week after the surgery, my arm with the graft started swelling, and I quickly took off my wedding ring as the swelling came all the way down to my fingers. I presented the swelling to the healthcare workers at convenient care, who quickly promoted me to the local emergency room at Carle Hospital. The doctor took one look and said, "Mr. Swinford, I'm calling Barnes hospital, and we are making arrangements to transfer you. This inflammatory response has caused a spike in your potassium level, and we are treating that and checking the blood flow. But your surgeons will need to see if any correction is indicated."

Ugh. Please, not another rough 200-mile ambulance ride. The medicines administered to lower the potassium caused me to feel loopy, so I couldn't put up much of an argument. I was wheeled into the ER in St. Louis at 5:00 a.m. Fortunately, it all checked out, and the graft did not have to be redone. This dialysis business was off to a shaky start, and I had not received my first treatment. And this unscheduled road trip left me a three-plus hour drive from home, and my wife did not drive in winter conditions.

"Roger, I'm in a bit of a pinch. I'm getting discharged from the hospital and need a ride home."

"No problem, Doug. Are you at Carle or OSF?"

"Well, that's the thing. I'm not in Urbana. I'm actually in St. Louis."

"Oh, wow, okay, let me talk to Jacque."

I worked with Roger Mcelroy for many years and was always friends with him and his wife, Jacque. I didn't know any other couple who lived out their Christian faith more than Roger and Jacque. When I hit my previous critical illness ruts, Roger was always reassuring with prayers and the general sense of, "Doug, it is going to be okay either way."

I always appreciated his dedication. The only wickedness in Roger was his sense of humor. In this instance, he just said, "I can come get you, and I won't charge as much as a taxi."

"I would hope not, Roger. After all, a taxi driver would probably be better company than you!"

"I would tend to agree with you, Doug, but I am bringing Jacque along."

"Oh great, in that case, I would expect to pay full fare." I knew just to stop there as I wasn't going to get ahead of Roger in satire, sarcasm, or any other response. It was a delightful ride home, and I appreciated their sacrificing a day to help me.

As the calendar turned to 2020, I went in to see Dr. Attia and have him see my new graft. "Let's see what you have there. Hmm. It is coming along but still going to be sore, but I have to start you on dialysis. Your GFR (glomerular filtration rate) is 9, and usually, we start treatment at 10-15. Low side of normal is 60. At your age, you would likely be 80 or over still if you weren't a transplant patient. The treatment will help get some of this edema off you and make your legs feel better. January 17 is your start date."

Before I could start, they made me attend a meeting. I took away a couple of main points. "1. You don't have to do this. 2. If you don't do this, you will die a natural death." *Okay, okay, I get it. I put it off as long as I could. Let's do it!*

I reported to dialysis like it was just another job that I had to do.

"Hi, my name is Dolly, and I'm going to get you started," the technician said. "I'm going to give you a smaller needle since this is your first treatment. We will have the doctor give you a prescription for lidocaine cream to put on your arm at home an hour before you come. Wrap it with Saran Wrap to help it soak in. It helps with the sting of the needles." She spoke pleasant enough, but the stick was bigger than what I was used to from the lab work or even an IV. Once in, though, I didn't really notice it.

My session lasted for three and a half hours. No breaks were planned. I feared I would need a bathroom break, but Dolly said they would disconnect me if required. I soon learned when an artificial kidney is pulling all the fluid out of your body, you don't have to worry about potty breaks. Instead, my concerns were cramps and occasional nausea. I didn't want to get up anyway because the clock stopped on the machine and just prolonged the treatment time.

One day, my stomach became so upset I asked to be unhooked. As one tech worked on my tubing to free me, I asked another to get a basin. "Let the treatment run. I'm not going to make the bathroom."

So, they put a little curtain up around me and gave me some privacy. From then on, I kept my little emergency basin and would ride out whatever might come. I learned to let the staff know if I wasn't feeling good, and they could adjust the machines to take less fluid off.

The whole treatment from arrival to when the needles came out and the bleeding stopped lasted about four and a half hours. Three times a week. Tough job, but I liked the compensation.

Walking into the dialysis clinic one spring morning, the air was kind, and the sun shined bright in a cloudless, blue sky. I thought, *I should just skip today. Pick up some Subway sandwiches, take my wife to nearby Homer Lake, and have a picnic. That would be a wonderful use of this glorious day.* I knew of other patients skipping a day here or there and getting by with it. Deep down, I knew I couldn't afford to be reckless. It was almost like a temptation for a particular sin that you knew you *really really* shouldn't indulge. I concluded that the idea needed to be left as just a flirtation and continued inside. It so happened to be an atypical day.

After the weigh-in and hook-up, I finished a memoir titled *Shirley Jones: A Memoir.* I bumped into the book on my Kindle. Recalling the *Partridge Family* show and one of my sisters having David Cassidy posters helped pique my interest, and it was a good read. Hour two, I sneaked a few pretzels and sipped a little water. Eating and drinking were discouraged since they could alter body chemistry. We had our own TV. I didn't particularly like game shows, but I caught on to 70s reruns of *Match Game.* I found it entertaining with Gene Rayburn and Richard Dawson hamming it up. Somewhere between Brett Somers trying to hit

Charles Nelson Reilly over the head with her card, I drifted off to sleep.

My phone rang, which wasn't that easy to hear with all the alarms on the machines blaring up and down the long rectangular room with 16-20 patients at a time. One of the nurses nudged me, "Mr. Swinford, your phone is ringing."

I answered sleepily, "Hello, this is Doug."

"Mr. Swinford, I'm calling from the Utility Employees Credit Union. We like to update customer information from time to time." I had forgotten about the account and couldn't recall any recent correspondence. Given I only remembered having about $40 in the account, I hadn't given it much thought. I gave the usual address and so on and almost hung up but decided to check the balance.

"Can you tell me the balance of the account?"

"Sure, Mr. Swinford. I see here that you have $8,495.22."

WHAT? I had her double-check.

"Yes, you had monthly deposits held from your check for several years. That is your balance."

This day was looking up.

A good book, fresh pretzels, cold water, a funny show, all capped off with a surprising windfall. *That* was a good day at dialysis!

Dialysis gets a bad rap. It should be called *live*-alysis. If only they had an equivalent to help out the liver like have for the kidneys. Like with anything else, we adapted. My wife cooked while I was at treatment since my time went over the lunch hour. "Honey, I'm baking fish dipped in panko and making rice."

In addition to the nutrition, my wife sensed that I needed something to look forward to during the long treatments. To keep my morale up, I would reflect on the anticipated fish, Italian beef, chicken and noodles, or whatever other culinary delights she made. A steady stream of healthy meals. I would eat when I came home and then nap. The treatment seemed to help the leg swelling during the first few months. Then in late April 2020, there was a turn of events.

"Mr. Swinford. Mr. Swinford, can you hear me?" It was Shalonda, the manager at CU Dialysis.

Patients often fell asleep, but in this case, I wasn't waking up when my treatment ended. I dreamt of being in a distant Arctic place when I finally regained consciousness. I was very confused. And cold. I was always cold at treatment. Shalonda looked so worried and asked if I needed a wheelchair. She also urged that we go to the ER. My wife gathered me up, and we headed home to figure out what to do. We knew the ER would transfer us on my frequent flyer long ambulance ride. We wanted Jessi to come over and help Lynne get me stabilized. In my semi-coherent state after leaving the facility, I told Lynne, "Rachel had a prescription for lactulose sent to Walgreens last week. I didn't think I needed it yet, but we need to pick it up."

My symptoms had all the appearances of poisons having built up in my system, and excess ammonia was causing the dreaded hepatic encephalopathy, which indicates end-stage liver disease. The slide changed from worry about being able to work, to losing more of my freedom with dialysis, to now fighting for my life. Again.

Chapter 13

Tangling with Eternity

My youngest daughter Rachel had graduated nursing school and departed for Florida, working as a liver transplant coordinator at Mayo Clinic in Jacksonville. Both of my daughters who were nurses followed my regular lab work, and Rachel had been urging my overseers at Barnes to start me on lactulose.

She called the evening of my mental confusion. "Dad, I don't know why, but your liver seems to be protesting you doing dialysis. Your liver numbers have edged worse and worse. I'm not surprised about what happened today. I talked to Dr. Crippin and Pam, and they faxed a prescription for you several days ago. Have you started it yet?"

I replied, "I'm sorry. I know I should have picked it up and started the lactulose, and maybe I wouldn't have gotten sick at treatment today. I didn't know how close I was to this kind of event. Now I'm just coming out of the murkiness and can walk again. Jessi and Lynne have given me the medicine, and we are now preparing for a late evening ride to Barnes." I wasn't eager to go, but it was obvious we had a marked change in my condition, and it was time for the transplant team to see what, if anything, they could do for me.

This mental confusion had not befallen me since the brief episode before my 2004 transplant, and I had been combative and out of my mind at that time. Now, when the symptoms came on, I was lethargic, often sleeping, and unable to think clearly. I had to take lactulose, which had the unpleasant effects of basically rinsing my system out to keep the ammonia level down.

So my new reality became stints in the hospital with occasional brief interludes at home—either Barnes or the local Carle Hospital for a few days at a time until I was able to clear my mind. In early May, when I was back home for a bit, Pam called from the transplant office and gave me some instructions. "Doug, we would like you to come, and we have a procedure to try and aid your liver efficiency."

Lynne and I headed down, hoping we could restore some function and get me out of this dreaded cycle. I had been losing days and was unable to recall what had happened. My daughters pushed me to stay hospitalized and get evaluated for a possible liver transplant. At any rate, the endoscopy-type procedure to help my liver ran into trouble when the doctors performing what was planned as outpatient surgery uncovered internal bleeding of a duodenal ulcer.

This event sent me in a spiral of being in and out of the ICU, trying to curb the bleeding and corral the mental confusion. Now I was too sick to do anything but try and stabilize and stay alive. With the latest blow, my kidneys failed completely and quit producing any urine. As we moved into June, my daughters pressed Barnes for answers and kept asking if I could be helped. Was a third liver transplant out of reach? The question had been asked six years prior, and I had been told it was not going to happen. Time had passed since then. Could a third transplant even be considered?

Rachel was no longer with Mayo as she moved away with her young son Everett and Army officer husband Kyle to Ft. Benning, Georgia. She had my records sent to surgeons at Mayo to give a second opinion She and Jessi made numerous calls and set up plans to take me on a road trip to Florida. At first, I was reluctant to have to go to another facility. Barnes wasn't perfect, but they had kept me going for many years. Rachel and Jessi had a sense of urgency, kept in close touch with the Barnes doctors, and made it clear we needed a decision regarding my status. My MELD (Model for End-Stage Liver Disease) score, the evaluating factor for qualifying for a transplant, was already very high.

I braced myself that this might be the end. I made my peace with God. I accepted my fate, whatever it may be. I had already survived way more than I ever thought that I could. I reminded myself that in 2004, I didn't think I could make it. Now, I needed to reach back and recall that maybe I could get through more than I thought. My kids advocated for me. Rachel called one night,

"Dad, I have a doctor at Mayo who says he will take your case if Barnes can't help you. This isn't over. We aren't giving up. This can be done, Dad!" She spoke with conviction, and I tried to believe. Hope, as expressed by my loved ones, was all that I had.

The old saying goes, "When it rains, it pours." My existing vision issue with macular degeneration now had an ongoing issue in my left eye with scrambled vision. I told Rachel one day on the phone, "Rachel, I really feel out of control. I can't think clearly; half of the time, I don't know where I am or what day it is. Now my vision is so distracted by what is going on in my left eye."

"I know, Dad, and Jessi and I have both tried to have an eye doctor from Barnes check you out since you have missed all of your appointments back home. I think there are just too many other issues to deal with, and your vision will have to wait. I'm sorry, Dad, we can't get you help."

Finally, between hospital stays, I was able to get a diagnosis and repair for a detached retina in the first week of July. Dr. Michael Tsipursky of our local Carle Clinic agreed to do the surgery despite my frail condition. It had gotten so bad that text messages I sent out would autocorrect some bizarre things and made reading my messages a real adventure in interpretation. I couldn't see well enough to discern my display.

On July 9, the committee at Barnes reviewed the tests of all my organ systems and decided to list me for a liver *AND* kidney transplant. A road trip to Florida was not necessary. The question remained if the call would come soon enough. I lay hospitalized in my local hospital the day I heard that Blue Cross had approved me, and I had a green light to get help. My local hospital released me on July 13, and the following day my wife and I were heading into the grocery store when we received the call that a donor was available. We were both stunned. We drove a few blocks, and Lynne said, "Honey, I can't drive to St. Louis. I'm too shaken. I'm excited, but I can't concentrate." She nearly ran a stop light.

"I would love to drive, but I can't see well enough. Just take it slow to home, and I'll call Jessi. I think they had a plan for this."

"Okay, Dad," Jessi said excitedly when I reached her. "I'll call Aaron and see if he can take you! And I will get ready and get the boys set up because I'm coming down to be with Lynne."

Jessi's husband, Tony, stayed behind with sons Vinny and Gio, in Springfield, Illinois. My son-in-law Aaron left Ashley and their children, Alton and baby Ayla, at home while he delivered Lynne and me to our destiny.

Here we go. As I recalled earlier, it was a sleepless night. Sleep wasn't necessary for me. It was a night for prayers, thoughts, and reflections. I had done my job. And I had given all my fortitude to survive the ravages of liver failure. The transplant team had done their part and decided sans partiality it was feasible to attempt a rare third liver replacement. I had my COVID test at about 9:00 p.m. That could be a deal breaker, but the night was quiet.

I entered the prep room at 4:40 a.m. I felt upbeat. Unless something went drastically wrong, I could only get better.

In contrast, I thought about the coin flip scene in the movie *No Country for Old Men*. The killer stood across from the gentleman at the rural gas station and did a coin flip. The elderly man wanted to know what they were flipping for. What was he going to win if he chose the right side that came up? The killer replied, "You stand to win everything." The tension in their conversation indicated a greater meaning; indeed, if the man chose the wrong side of the coin, he would be killed. He correctly chose heads, and the killer congratulated him, and the strain on the man's face released.

In my case, heads would be a restoration of health and potential release from dialysis. Tails would represent PSC and her fatal wares collecting their prize. But if I didn't choose the flip, I was likely down to days or weeks of survival, and not pleasant ones at that.

One of the female surgeons stood beside my bed and looked over my condition. My belly and legs were all grotesquely out of shape due to the extra 30 pounds of water I was carrying. On the door was a magnetic sign that indicated go or no go. It still said go for me, but I knew there could always be a last-minute problem discovered with the donor. Trying to make small talk with the surgeon, I said, "Well, the donor must be okay. I see we are a go."

She replied flatly while gently pressing down on my belly, "I'm not worried about the donor."

Oh no, I thought. *Could I be turned away at the last minute?* Nothing had gone right so far. Several nurses had already tried to get my IV started to no avail. My right arm looked and felt badly beaten from numerous lab sticks and IVs from my hospitalizations over the last three months. My left arm teased with decent veins, but the dialysis graft in my upper arm made it off-limits. One of the nurses came in and looked at my arm and threw her hands up, and said, "I'm not touching that. There isn't anything to work with." She marched right out of the room.

The surgeon left, and now my "Coach" from several weeks prior entered.

"Why isn't Mr. Swinford's IV in yet? It is almost 6:30. He should be ready!" Her disgust was evident as she grabbed the ultrasound machine to take matters into her own hands. This was my first experience with heightened tensions between staff members and raised voices. Prep rooms were usually very methodical.

Even so, I learned to get used to things not going to plan at my work. Construction jobs, or emergency response to cut gas lines, rarely went to design, and the venting and language sailed along the lines of sailors and sots. This was tea and crumpets by comparison.

Dr. Kahn, protégé of Dr. Chapman and the lead surgeon on this case, entered and implored the staff that I needed to be in the OR in 30 minutes. He was upbeat and wasn't surprised in the least by my poor condition. He patted my arm as he said, "We will get you fixed up."

I spoke to Coach. "Am I okay here? Are we going to be able to do this? The other surgeon seemed very concerned about my condition."

"Douglas, do you recall me telling you this would be difficult and would have setbacks? This is just the beginning. But we brought you down here to transplant you, and that is about to happen." Coach had already proven prophetic, and her predictions would continue to come true.

Again, Coach reassured me, and despite my pummeled arm and not knowing how much punishment I would get before the big sleep, I felt reflective and thought of scripture to meditate upon.

I was thinking of Psalm 23: "The Lord is my shepherd, I shall not want. He makes me lie down in green pastures. He leads me beside still waters, he restores my soul. Though I walk through the valley of the shadow of death, I shall fear no evil..."

I had trouble recalling the whole psalm but ran through what I could remember. Doing so helped me stay calm about the continued futile efforts at an IV. I understood that it was required to be placed prior to my entering the operating room. Time slipped past the time the doctor said we needed to go, and I no longer looked at my arm or what they had done. In exasperation, Coach finally placed a makeshift tourniquet on my arm, and we wheeled down the hall to the operating room where a team member immediately started working on a control line in the area of my collarbone. He covered my face and told me, "We usually wait to put these in after you are sedated, but we don't think that IV is viable. Bear with me, and I will give you several lidocaine shots."

They covered my face with blue paper, and I lay very still. The female surgeon who had expressed concern about my condition assumed I was sedated already and said, "I'm really not looking forward to this one!"

One of the staff instantly spoke out, "Doctor, the patient is still awake."

It was very quiet for a few seconds, and I said, "It's okay. You can knock me out with a hammer if necessary!"

The staff all laughed except for the surgeon who made the comments. I took no offense. I knew I was a hot mess.

After the chuckle, things seemed to fall into place. I was asked what kind of music I wanted to hear, and I requested Hawaiian-type music similar to what my wife listened to while hula dancing. I was most concerned about her. She adamantly assured me that I would sail through this, while my daughters were more guarded and had been through this before.

I listened to the music and relaxed. With the control line in, a flurry of activity went on around me. They put a mask on me and instructed me to breathe in deeply. I was fed the milk of amnesia. I glanced at the clock and it was 8:20 a.m. As I fell asleep, I expected to wake up that evening, similar to my other surgeries. But this rebuild was a bigger job, so I was in for the longest snooze of my life.

I clawed myself to the finish line, and the team began their work. My wife and daughter Jessica stood by at the Parkway Hotel connected just off the northeast side of the massive Barnes-Jewish Hospital complex. With the pandemic, there were no surgical waiting rooms with tense family members, but my closest support team waited just a short walk away.

At 4:45 p.m., Dr. Kahn spoke with my daughter and wife and explained that the new liver was in, but I had lost a lot of blood, and they had difficulty stabilizing me. They had hoped to complete the liver and kidney, but I needed time in the ICU to try and stabilize and dialyze me. The team could rest up. Jessica recalls Dr. Kahn sounding a bit weary. Lynne was allowed to see me in the ICU that night, but I was never conscious, and my abdomen was not closed up all the way. Material covered the open wound, and I was intubated along with an attachment to my neck connected to the dialysis machine. This was going to go into at least tomorrow.

The team called at 5:00 a.m. and reported that I had stabilized in the night, and they went back to work. And the phone rang again at 9:30 a.m.

Jessica answered, "Hi, this is Jessi."

Dr. Kahn responded, "Well, we started with a thorough look at the liver, and the blood flow was excellent, and organ looked good, so we closed it up. Then we put the kidney in. He is all done." Dr. Kahn sounded much more confident. "He is off dialysis, and blood pressure has stabilized. He is still heavily sedated and will remain closely observed."

One of the effects of anesthesia is amnesia, and that feature was certainly effective for me. I heard from a nurse that perhaps I had raised a bit of a ruckus in the ICU. I don't know how I could go about that because I was intubated, but maybe I was thrashing about or trying to get up. I had no recollection. After my glance at the clock the morning they started in, I didn't remember a thing until the morning of Friday, July 17. I woke in a dimly lit room with no one around. When the nurse came in, I asked, "What day is it?"

"Oh, it's Friday," she responded.

I remarked, "I've never been asleep that long before!" My legs felt like rubber, and my first concern was if I could walk.

I began a systems check and felt quite pleased. I didn't seem to have any overwhelming pain, just more numbness. I had learned, though, that the raw pain was a day or two down the road when the anesthesia and big jolt of steroids wore off a bit. Still, there was enough of an edge that I accepted the Dilaudid or Oxycodone they offered me. Early in my transplant career, I would try and "tough it out" with minimal pain meds. Forget that. If something helped me, I was taking it.

I was on the complete side of the surgery. Was the hard part behind or still ahead?

CHAPTER 14

LADY IN THE WHITE DRESS

As the hours went by, I found pain when I tried to move. I wanted and needed to walk. The first few days, I had so many accouterments that it was only with the help of two people that I could muster a few steps. The physical and occupational therapists were so helpful as they taught me the best way to do things I had done with ease for my whole life, like getting out of bed. Simple, right? Not after major abdominal surgery. I had heard women talk of the pain of C-section surgery, and now I felt something similar. The abdominal wall is so central to the body. I had to roll and pitch just right. Every time I had to get up or make a major move, I cursed under my breath.

But we had two big jobs done. The donated liver and kidney were managing in their new environment so far. The first week, I had a vancomycin-resistant enterococcus infection. I received treatments for it, and yet, I was having almost daily tests "looking" for it or, maybe more specifically, trying to find out how it was affecting my heart and other organs, if at all. I knew that I would have to feel worse before I felt better. Mostly, I felt numb and sore and had very little appetite.

On the good side, I was enjoying the return of visions of the night sky while in my hazy state under pain meds. I had a splendid view of brilliant lights flashing like fireworks. And the stars and constellations hung like figures from a baby's mobile. I was not just looking at the sky; I was *in* the sky! I tried to draw a line to connect the Big Dipper, but my arm would tire. The Milky Way acted as a subtle headband across the sky. All this activity was a welcome escape from the full awareness of this difficult leg of the journey.

During the first week post-transplant and after getting to a regular room, I could get a visitor a day during set hours. My wife and three girls came, and this was a huge lift for my spirits. The malaise went into the second week, and I knew I wasn't going home in nine days like after my second transplant. I did acquire another visitor who was in my room when I didn't have company.

She wore a long white dress. She appeared to be elderly, maybe along the lines of my mother, who couldn't visit because she was in a nursing home herself. Anyway, the lady kept to herself. She stood near the door, leaning against the wall. I was going to ask the nurses about her, but I figured they would just say, "Now, Mr. Douglas, don't you know you are seeing things? You have had a lot of medication." Fine, whatever, but I know I saw her, and it was not a dream. Could she be an angel? Or a soul collector of some kind? I certainly wasn't out of the woods yet. Like with my dreams and visions, I found her comforting. I never felt afraid of her or that she meant any harm. Her role seemed to be observation.

Toward the end of July, Dr. Jenny Yu and Dr. Chapman started discussing my release. Dr. Jenny and her team saw me every day. I felt an advocate in Dr. Jenny. She would give me the next goal to get to and listen to my woes. I looked forward to seeing her every day.

Now, as to my release, it was a *conditional release*. I would be required to stay very close to the hospital for several weeks. Jessica had helped Lynne move from the *Parkway Hotel,* which was in the process of going through an acquisition, and moving to a less expensive Airbnb where she would have a kitchen to work with.

As I prepared to get out two weeks post-transplant, they had taken all my drains out except one. And it was a nuisance, located on my upper right leg, right in my belt area, a couple of inches below my kidney incision. It had one of those little hand grenade-size collectors, but that wasn't the problem. Where the drain went into my body wasn't stitched tightly, and all the clear excess fluid was looking for places to leak out. So I had to have endless bandaging and gown changes to stay dry. "Can't we take this thing out?" I pleaded.

"No, it is serving a purpose and working as intended," was the consistent reply.

My coordinator Pam Thurston helped work out our details with continued treatment and follow-ups. We didn't have our own car there, so a taxi was provided for the short ride to the Airbnb. Usually, I was excited to get out of the hospital, but not this time. I had no strength, energy, or appetite, and I was in existence mode, which is generally tolerated better in a hospital setting.

I hated the Airbnb. For one, I wasn't very comfortable yet and didn't feel that well. Lynne and Jessi ordered some food through Door Dash and put a plate of spaghetti in front of me, but nothing tasted good. The rooms were tired, old, stale-smelling converted apartments, and it did not have the comfort the newly renovated hotel offered. It was short of squalor, but if there was a Feng Shui rating, this was zip. Zero.

Lynne had to help with regular dressing and gown changes throughout the night. I slept in fits and starts. The nearby fire station ran calls at all hours. The TV had no regular news, only streaming services. I was mostly grouchy because I didn't feel good, and on the second day, I woke up with a fever.

They checked me at the outpatient clinic, but nothing beyond the typical post-surgery woes appeared to be present, and my fever subsided. The next day, I woke up with chest pains. I called my daughters, and they said to go to the emergency room *NOW!*

The emergency room entrance was only a quarter mile away. I dialed up an Uber, and a young man delivered us promptly. The staff saw my condition and sent me right to triage. Within an hour, I learned I had a massive infection and would need to undergo surgery. My first thought was, *Damnit, I just learned how to get out of bed without it hurting so bad, and I'm going to have to start all over again.*

Why did Coach, who predicted all of the trouble I would encounter, have to be so damned right? I underwent a double transplant successfully and prayed it would be gradually better. Not so fast. After my infection "wash out" surgery, I woke up to all manner of unpleasant news. For starters, I couldn't talk because I was intubated. I was incredulous. What the hell was going on? I coughed fiercely most of the night. If I coughed hard enough, it set off an alarm, and a nurse would come and suction me so that I could breathe.

I had encountered numerous travails, but I had never been intubated with minimal sedation. Crazy thoughts rushed through my mind about the complaints I would levy for being in this situation and wanted to write a letter to the editor at *the St. Louis Post-Dispatch* about the inhumane treatment of patients. PETA would not stand for such treatment of animals, and here I was choking with a damned tube down my throat. I couldn't talk or see, and my call button was always out of reach. I just felt helpless. The effects of infection and another surgery were a cocktail I wouldn't wish on anyone. I needed help!

Early the next morning came Dr. Jenny. I felt delighted to see her. She would set this straight. "Mr. Swinford, I know this is uncomfortable, but we have kept the vent in for now as we may need to take you back to surgery soon." Then I found that the vent was the least of my concerns.

Dr. Jenny continued, "The infection was traumatic for your new organs, and there was so much swelling that we couldn't close the incision due to the inflammation of the liver."

I listened but kept waving for pen and paper, which her team provided. I wrote, "Tube out?"

My right hand had an IV, and my scribble was barely legible.

Dr. Jenny replied, "I'll talk to Dr. Chapman about the vent. It is important right now to keep it placed. It is difficult to put back in again, and we aren't sure when we are taking you back into surgery. Now the kidney team is going to come in and start dialysis to try and help save your kidney."

I don't know if I have had a lower point in my long journey of fighting liver disease and scrapping to stay alive. I was terribly uncomfortable. My abdomen remained open and had some type of wound pump, and my old and new organs were very sick from this infection. Would all of the work the team put in go for naught? It had been a valiant effort to save me. There are limits to the human body and what can be done. Perhaps we had reached it.

There was a bright spot that day. My oldest daughter Ashley was in to see me. I kept trying to scribble notes. I tried to find some way to joke or make light of the situation. Ashley helped her son Alton make heartfelt videos imploring me to get better. Their encouragement made me feel better, and Rachel flew in from Georgia. Given my perilous condition, it appeared that COVID rules were set aside, as later, my wife and Jessi came through for short visits.

I worked on a note with Ashley's help. "Dr. Chapman, can you please have this tube removed? I had been motioning to the staff about it, and they said it took a doctor's order to take it out." Also, I couldn't get too animated, or they would put those cursed "boxing gloves" on. The gloves weren't as terrible as the vent, but very frustrating in that I couldn't use my hands for anything.

That evening, the esteemed Dr. Chapman came in. I gestured about the tube. He glanced at my scribbles, but he knew what I was wanting. He explained, "Doug, we will have to get you closed up at some point. I would hate to send you home with a wound pump. I'm keeping the vent in as a precaution and will take it out as soon as we can."

I waived my arms and implied I couldn't take it anymore.

"Just hang in there." As he walked out, I knew he sensed my frustration. But he was experienced and knew his job was to try and get me through this alive, and my comfort at this critical time was secondary. I had always held him in such high regard, but then I felt furious at him. It goes without saying, I had been through a couple of really bad days. I hoped the military term of FUBAR was not applicable here. My family and I still clung to hope.

Chapter 15

Turning Point, August 5

A team may be flailing in a sporting contest, like a basketball game, with nothing going right. But a player steals the ball and makes a layup, changing the momentum of the entire game. Then the team rallies. In my dire circumstances following surgery to deal with the infection, I was in an appalling condition. With my new organs irritated and failing, the huge incision had to be left open. I couldn't take any nourishment outside of IV fluids for the time being.

Dr. Jenny came, and all my fight to advocate for myself was gone. I just laid there, still unable to talk, and listened. I needed a big play; I needed something good to happen.

"Doug," she started. "We have discussed the situation and decided that it will be a few days before we can attempt to close you up. So we are going to take the vent out and will just have to place it in again when we go back to the operating room. Anesthesia will come and remove it. After that, we will address getting some nutrition and will try and place a feeding tube."

Dr. Jenny made the big play. I was elated. The vent coming out was like an elephant had one foot on my chest, and then it was lifted. I felt so relieved. Now for some nutrition. I didn't care if it was a feeding tube. I just knew that my body needed help. I couldn't remember the last time I had anything to eat. I guessed at the Airbnb, but even then, I was nibbling.

Just a few hours after the vent came out, I went to a procedures room for a resident to place my feeding tube. I wished for more sedation as I heard his overseer coaching him on what to do. They could watch on a camera, and I didn't think they knew how aware I was of what was happening. He kept trying and failing to get the tube placed right. I wanted the instructor to take over, but this sounded like a test. The young man did his best, but after repeatedly gagging me as the tube came back up my throat, they withdrew and conceded that, for whatever reason, this procedure failed.

But hey, we had plan B. They placed an intravenous feeding tube and got some nutrition going. My youngest daughter Rachel came in later that day, and I was feeling a whole lot better about life. I could breathe freely, and I could talk. I was still on dialysis, and the staff told my daughters that the liver was recovering. It might just turn out that the liver was successful, but I might have to continue dialysis.

That evening, Dr. Jenny came in at about 8:00 p.m. to change the dressing on my open wound. I was amazed at her working hours because she was often the first person I saw in the morning. Getting on Dr. Chapman's team was difficult, so I knew Dr. Jenny was very dedicated. She began to work with great precision.

She had the dressing off and said, "Doug, would you like to see your new liver?"

I had a hard time imagining that the right side of my incision was open. How was it not bleeding? I guess it had to do with the covering and the wound pump. I glanced down enough to see the dark red. I was afraid to move too much. In hindsight, I should have handed Dr. Jenny my phone and requested a picture for the sake of curiosity. It's not every day that your new organ is on display.

I asked the doctor, "So, where did you grow up?"

She replied, "In a small town in Indiana."

We chatted freely, as it took about 45 minutes to complete the work. She kindly offered me some pain medicine because there was some pressure applied to the area. I enjoyed the conversation and the careful work she handled. In terms of my mental state, I turned a corner that day. Once again, I felt that I could come through this. After Coach had done her best to prepare me, Dr. Jenny gave me a calm confidence that this would work out.

Chapter 16

Motor Home Escape

After a few stable days, Dr. Chapman came by on August 8 and explained, "Doug, we are going to try and close up the wound and remove the wound pump. The kidney team tells us your kidney seems to be rebounding, and you are off dialysis."

"Will this be a lesser surgery than the others?" I asked.

"It should be. We will see how it goes."

I could only imagine the scene in the operating room. "Okay, you two push the skin together, and I'll sew it shut!"

I didn't know how they would perform this task, and I didn't ask. I recall the wound being two or three inches wide when Dr. Jenny had to change the bandage. I hoped this new liver rebounded enough from the swelling to allow trained hands to cover it again. I thought of the trauma to this liver and kidney over the last few weeks.

These organs previously resided in a healthy, vibrant individual just a few weeks ago—laughing, crying, eating, and drinking—

a fellow traveler wading through life. I don't know if it was fate or destiny, but a life-ending calamity occurred. I had no way of knowing what had happened to them. When all of this was behind me, I could write a letter of gratitude to the family, and I hoped they would respond. The only thing I knew about them was that when the call came that this donor was considered high-risk due to intravenous drug use.

Perhaps a troubled soul, but the only other hint we had was that the doctor implied to my daughters that the organs were pristine. This may have indicated a younger person.

Antibiotics, given for specific bacteria, shot down their targets like an incoming asteroid on a video game. With the assistance the liver complied and was able to be secured. Maybe, just maybe, the tempestuous quest for harmony could be actualized. The carefully sewn-in instruments of life were saved from the grave and now involved a symbiotic joining. I depended on them, and they on me. And while this donor had passed, they were a hero in death, to me and likely others as well.

After a couple of days, I started to hear rumblings about my going to a rehabilitation facility. My mind immediately thought of the facility my mother had been in, and I thought, *Oh no!* My recollections were of very elderly people sitting in wheelchairs and nodding off.

I sarcastically told my wife, "So, do I have any say in this rehab thing? I'm not too keen on it."

She replied, "But, honey, you can't walk; you can't take care of yourself."

"Okay, I'll agree to two days. But if I don't like it, I'm going home!"

My transplant coordinator Pam came by and discussed with my wife what center I would be sent to. She and my wife agreed on the Rehabilitation Institute of St. Louis, located just down the street. As it so happened, Coach stopped by briefly before my discharge and wished me good luck.

"I appreciate everything you have done for me, Coach."

She just smiled at the name I had given her and walked out.

I was not sure of my status and still felt a little confused. Had I slipped down too far? My cognitive function remained lacking. I kept repeating myself like I had been sitting on a bar stool drinking beer all day. I kept losing track of my phone. As I was often isolated due to COVID, my phone was my lifeline. I could receive video messages from family, so I was frantic, like a kid looking for their blanky when it was misplaced.

"Mr. Swinford, your phone is right under your pillow. No need to worry," my nurse would say.

I was scattered, and the question was, had the poisons of disease rendered a toll that was not recoverable?

I had never been a patient in a rehab facility before. Previous surgeries and setbacks had never left me so broken down. And I was 60 years old, not 31 or 44 like the previous reconstructions.

And it wasn't just age; it was also the length of downtime. In the last three months, I had been in the hospital for all but a handful of days. Many of those days, I remained confined to my bed. And so my life experience was now adding rehab to the list of unwanted but necessary adventures.

My first challenge was learning the director's name at the facility. Dr. Husky had come by in her wheelchair and introduced herself. During my stay, she came to say "hi" almost daily. Right away, she explained how she had come by her last name. She had attended a meeting, spied a man she found interesting, and asked who he was. She was told, "That is Dr. Husky."

She said, "Well, I like what I see, and I like the name. I'm going to marry that man! And I did."

Right off, I could tell she was feisty, and I respected her. Her wheelchair spoke to me that *her path had not been easy*. Just so happened, it was my current method of transport as well. I came here to hopefully discard my wheels and resume on my own. Her visits had a purpose, and I didn't perceive that a significant part of my rehab would be cerebral. She loved to come in and say, "Do you remember my name?"

I thought, *Oh, hell, it's a dog breed. Is it a boxer?* "Doctor, I can't quite recall your name this morning, but if you remind me, I'll get it next time."

"Ha, ha. That's okay. You are a little foggy yet, and transplants are tough business. But we will work with you with physical, speech, and occupational therapy to get you shaped up!"

Dr. Husky was executing an agenda with her visits. What was my physical and mental condition? How could she best inspire me? She conveyed a force of will, such that if a bull was charging down the hallway, she could square up with him in her chair and stop him dead cold. There was no room for failure here.

I told Dr. Husky, "Doctor, you remind me of my Uncle Ed Gerstner. Little Eddie had polio as a child. His 11 siblings, including my mom, Barbie, rallied around little Eddie. His affliction didn't stop him from *anything*. Plucky by nature, he still played basketball in high school, still got the best girl, Aunt Carlyne, and was successful in business. He has the most remarkable spirit of love and kindness."

"Mr. Douglas, I like hearing about your family because you seem clearer in your thinking about them."

After she left, I thought that while not always visible by limp or wheelchair, life deals a tough hand to us all.

I was inspired by both Dr. Husky and my Uncle Ed, but I was in my own fix. I'm sure I could have looked on Facebook or Instagram and found some lofty platitudes about overcoming adversity. That type of notion wouldn't mean a damned thing to me, though. My belly hurt. My drain leaked. I had a pounding headache, and as my former Pastor John Sims liked to say with a grin, "Sucks to be you!"

The first evening at rehab, the nurse gave me a schedule for the next day.

"Nurse, is this right? I have three appointments tomorrow?"

"Why do you ask, Mr. Douglas? Do you have other plans?" she said curiously.

"Yes, actually, I do. I planned to start training for a marathon."

Without hesitation, she fired back, "Well, you are in the right place because the last I checked, you have to be able to walk before you can run, and right now, you can't even get out of bed by yourself! Don't even try it. If you fall, both of us are going to be in trouble. Use that call button! And clear your schedule for tomorrow because your plans will have to wait!"

The sun crept through the blinds to announce a new day, my first full day. Outside, it was the dog days of August. Hot and steamy. Before I could review my thoughts and shake off the fitful sleep, a nurse slipped in to take my blood pressure. "You will need to try and eat some breakfast, as your therapist will be here soon for your first appointment." She grabbed a container off my tray and started shaking it. "If nothing else, try and drink this Ensure."

I had food now but scant appetite. The old cliché is that man can't live on bread alone and sure as hell can't live on Ensure. I picked around and ate a piece of toast. The door opened, and at first, I thought it was one of my daughters. With my vision impaired and so many of the staff being millennials as my kids were, this happened often. Then I heard her talk and knew it was a therapist. "Okay, Mr. Swinford, I have read your chart. We have a plan to help get you back on your feet. We will get you down to the therapy room and get started."

We entered the sprawling workout room. This was a far cry from the facility my mom had been in. Windows wrapped around, giving a bright, cheerful effect. At Mom's place, the patients were there mainly because they were wearing out with old age. Here, the cruelties of life were visible across all age spectrums with many young people. Was it car accidents or falls? I didn't know, but for a young person to be here meant it was significant—life-changing for some. I guessed there were more stroke and heart attack patients in my age group. I empathized with all of them as we were all in a hell of a fight against pain, loss of balance, and mental acuity. Dignity was at stake. Could we regain it? Would we ever be productive members of society after all of this, whatever *this* was?

"Now, Douglas, I want you to head for the other end and go as far as you can."

I wobbled along on my walker, and when I got too shaky, she steadied me with the belt around my waist and had me turn around. I got a rest when I returned back to my starting place. *Wow,* this was harder than digging a ditch back in the gas department at work. After the physical work, she explained as she motioned with her hand. "Now, Douglas, we will have you work on a series of puzzles and games." Some were shapes and things you learned as a child, but I had to work to figure even the simplest problems out. What I was unable to do was tell myself that this facility was exactly where I needed to be.

Back in my private room, an occupational therapist was waiting to do an evaluation.

"Mr. Swinford, I would like you to draw a clock face and place the hands at 4:15." I was already beat from physical therapy, but I took my best shot at it. The therapist smiled and beamed, "That's very good, Douglas. We can try that again soon. And as your hands get steadier, it will make it easier for you."

The therapist's personality was over the top kind and made me feel good as I relaxed and dozed off, exhausted. When I woke, the lady in the white dress was back! I thought for sure she was just an observer at Barnes-Jewish, but here, she stood in the same place across from the restroom, just minding her business. She never looked directly at me or spoke. Her posture and what I could see of her features suggested a motherly vibe. She was concerned but not actively involved in my care. If she was a spiritual being, she was undercover since she bore no wings or radiant glow. I saw no indication that I was still in imminent danger of dying, so the soul collector idea I had entertained during her presence at the hospital didn't seem to mesh either. Her presence offered a sense of solace, almost like she was a stand-in for my mother. And Mom, still in skilled nursing due to her moderate dementia, was unable to come to me.

After lunch, I dozed off again and saw my wife sitting next to the bed when I woke up. I started talking to her, but she didn't respond. I dozed off again, and then she was gone.

When she came later, I asked, "Were you here earlier because I tried talking, and you didn't say anything?"

"No," she said, then explaining her lodging changes.

"Okay, well, I don't see her right now, but have you seen the lady in the white dress standing by the door?"

"What lady?" my wife replied.

"Oh, never mind, it's just a lady that has been coming in the room, just like guarding the door. I saw her at the hospital a couple of times."

My wife laughed. "I think you are seeing things!"

The next day, I was surprised to see my sister Cheryl there when I woke up. "Hi, sis; when did you come down from Battle Creek?"

She didn't answer. After closing my eyes for a few minutes, I didn't see her anymore. Later that day, after a nap, I saw my dad! Dad had passed away several years ago. He had a fixed but happy gaze, and I knew then that *I had definitely been seeing things.*

The therapy was much more comprehensive than I had envisioned. I knew the staff were helping me, so I had no gripes at rehab. The staff was patient and not surprised by any of my struggles. The most persistent issue had been the leaky drain.

"Nurse, I'm sorry, but I'm going to need a dressing change and a fresh gown."

"Again? You change clothes more often than my teenage daughter."

I didn't have a good comeback for that. Despite my attempts at witty banter, I remained slow to come up with good retorts. Dr. Husky was still able to get me on her quiz. I might get her name right proudly, and then she would ask what day it was. I was starting to grasp that when I had so much sickness, surgery, more surgery, and a barrage of painkillers, my brain became sick and needed to heal, too.

Eventually, I could start sending my plate back with less food. I expected any day that I would see a workman wheel in a dolly with a 55-gallon drum of Ensure, and the staff could pump it directly into a cup for me. I'm sure so many of my unused bottles labeled for me were crowding the fridge that the nurses had no place for their lunch.

I know I had heard it over and over. "Mr. Swinford, for your recovery, we need to get your protein level up."

To avoid the lecture, I started raising my bottle of said drink as a toast when a staffer came in. "Cheers! Do you care to join me?"

One nurse came back with a flat retort, "Hardy, har-har, Mr. Douglas. We are just trying to help you get more calories!"

They were getting tired of me.

Jessica called one day during my lunch break and said, "Dad, I want to come down and visit. Tony is working surgery today, but Steve and Sheryl will help with the boys. I already checked with the staff, and they said you can have a visitor."

"Great, Jessi! I can't wait to see you. Tell your in-laws how much I appreciate their help."

She drove the 100 miles and bounded into the room with a bag in hand. "Dad, I brought your favorite snacks! Snickers, Fritos, some mints, and Twizzlers."

"Thanks, Jessi. I'll choose some of that over this minestrone soup anytime!"

From the start of the whole ordeal in May, during my inpatient hospitalizations, Jessi saw to my culinary needs by supplementing my cafeteria grub using *Door Dash,* usually from the nearby Applebee's. And having been an ICU nurse herself, she always included a treat for the staff of chocolate cake or a variety of food items they could share. The nursing staff assisted in this caper since they had retrieval duties. Jessi worked every angle to try and get me more comfortable and try to entice my appetite.

Jessi was upbeat and eager to talk, "Dad, I can't wait to tell you about the GoFundMe. I put up your picture as the 'Transplant Trooper' on Facebook. I was shocked at how many people wanted to help. We met the goal quickly, and I believe it is going over."

"Wow, Jessi, I don't know what to say!"

I had been reluctant to post anything on social media, but Facebook was an excellent avenue to centralize information and allow friends to help if they so desired. The saga was long and drawn out, and I depended on my kids to handle inquiries, as Lynne could only keep in touch with a few close friends. If anyone called, I often couldn't find or reach the phone. I loved to text, but even after my recent retina repair, I could produce a word like "Zyzzyballuba" from the old *Pee-Wee's Playhouse* show.

I was sleeping fair at night, and about the third night, I had quite an "adventure." A large television screen stood in the middle of my private room. We had small televisions near the bed, but this big screen was for monitoring. Well, one night, as I drifted off, I was thinking about food. I wanted to go out to Bunny's Tavern in Urbana, Illinois. Their food was far superior to the hospital's bland diet and protein drinks. I could get a juicy cheeseburger and fries. Looking at the big screen, I saw it was a camera, and I could drive the room like a large motor home. I arrived at the bar, which was a stretch since it was 200 miles away in Illinois, but I was thinking big.

I nearly fell while going up a few stairs to go in the back way. Getting in the back door, I found that they had constructed an area for patrons who drank too much to lay down and sleep it off. Fortunately, there was an open bed next to other snoring customers because I was exhausted from the short walk. I rested a bit, then had to head back without even ordering food. I had to get to my *Motor Home.* I was so scared of the trouble I would be in if the nurses came to check on me and I wasn't there. What would Dr. Husky say? I better get back *now*! At some point, I woke up and was relieved to be back in my room. Nothing amiss; no one alarmed. *Whew.*

The next night, I met my friend Rick from rural Philo, Illinois, at Bunny's and again took a bed in the back room, but he brought me a steak dinner and fries. He took part in the raucous party in the main bar but checked on me in the resting area from time to time. One of the nurses from rehab was moonlighting as a waitress, and I borrowed some money from her. I needed to be sure to remember to pay her back.

When I left the bar, I couldn't find the motor home. *I've done it now!* But when I woke up, thank God, I was right in my room, and my bed alarms had not tripped off. With the dream feeling real, I asked the next morning if my lender nurse was working. I would have to get some money from my wife to pay her back!

What was going on here? This activity seemed to result from my brain bathing in excess amounts of ammonia, various pain meds, and anesthesia in a vicious cycle of lather, rinse, and repeat. No surprise, I experienced many short circuits. Pleasant dreams and non-threatening hallucinations brought welcome distractions from the ongoing trials of healing.

Dr. Husky operated her joystick to control her chair as she came in to see me after my therapy a few weeks into treatment.

"I see you are able to get around on your walker. I'm pleased with your progress. I'm going to discuss a discharge plan with the staff. Keep up the good work, and we can get you headed home soon."

Lynne headed home to check on the house, but more importantly, her daughter Amber neared term to deliver her first child. Madilyn Grace Bailey came safe and sound on August 24, 2020. My daughters had given us five grandchildren, and Madi put us at six. Amber lived close by to us and could keep an eye on the house, and she worked in my office at Ameren and could provide a few updates to co-workers.

My sister Cheryl offered help, so when I knew discharge was imminent, I requested that she come and claim me. Real this time, she drove down from Battle Creek, Michigan. Her late husband, Ray, was always so understanding to let her come to my aid. She had left him and their young kids at a wedding party to see me before my first transplant in 1991. In 2004, the kids and I had been sent home without a new liver, only to receive a call again the next day, and she was there to take me back to the hospital. Now, if my appointment at Barnes went okay on August 31, she was coming to get me safely home.

At the appointment, the nurse said, "Okay, sir, we are going to get that drain out!" It was as if someone had told me I had won the lottery. "You may want to wiggle your toes as this comes out. I will cut the stitch first. Are you ready?"

"Yes, let's do it!"

The nurse removing the drain looked like a fisherman pulling in a trot line. She just kept pulling and pulling as I wiggled my toes.

"There it is. I'll apply some pressure now."

"Oh, thank God!" I said as I put my head down and shook it with a chuckle. We were really getting somewhere now. The faucet leaked for 51 days and helped me lose 30 pounds, and I could actually put some comfortable sweatpants on. Goodbye, soaked gowns!

Cheryl and I headed out the next day for home on September 1, 2020. The whole saga started at work on the same date 37 years earlier.

Chapter 17

The Rock Keeps Rolling

On the ride home, I reminisced about what we had come through. And how we did it.

"Cheryl, that weekend in June when you brought Mom down and we had the get-together with the kids was amazing. What a lift for me, and then the parade my friends set up came the next day. What a morale boost."

I paused for a few minutes, then continued, "Comments made by several of my co-workers stayed with me. When I told them I was on the list for transplant again, I could still hear Bob Bell saying with certainty, 'If anyone can do it, you can!' And Les Storm commenting, 'You seem to have the ability to adapt to whatever is needed.' Bob and Les, and their spouses Lori and Stacy, had provided tremendous support to Lynne and me during the gut-wrenching time in and out of the hospital. If Bob and Les thought it was a lost cause, their tone would have been different." Cheryl just listened as I continued.

"In my precarious condition, I had a keen sense for genuine

comments. Veda Cooling, with connections at work and St. Joseph United Methodist church, assured me that Dottie and the prayer warriors were doing their best to lift me up just as they had in 2004."

Cheryl allowed me to continue to unwind my thoughts as we cruised down the road.

And as we pulled into the driveway, I saw the "Welcome home, Doug!" signs still in front of the house left from the June 20 parade that our go-getter friends, Kathy and Ruthie, arranged.

The COVID-friendly parade had been staged after a long stint in Barnes during the May to June period. Great timing to see everyone since I was back in the hospital a few days later. But that lovely day, I sat in the driveway and felt exhilarated and waved as cars and trucks went by honking and waving. And many friends stopped and visited.

Now the signs provided the "welcome home," once again.

At the June parade, it had been just a hope and a dream that one day I could get whole again and go back to Chris and Kathy's downstairs Shangri-La, *The Storm Cellar*. I wasn't kidding myself that day. The appreciation I felt was profound; at the time, it seemed more likely that it would be the last time I would ever see any of them. The gesture and the care shown were another push to help me through what seemed to be the suburbs of hell.

Having been in the clutches of death several times, I wish I could report the brilliance and wonder of the near-death experiences that others report. Perhaps, I haven't been as far down that road as to enter that realm. I never had to be shocked back to life. So, I can't say. All I know is that I understand there can come a level of discomfort for living that makes letting go more acceptable. I've learned it doesn't matter how I feel. I *wanted* to keep living, but with the weariness I felt, I prepared to die. It was for God to tip the scales. Even in the lowest moments, I sensed great power in the love and prayers of others. It was like a great tug-o-war between life and death. Too weak to pull on the rope myself, my friends and loved ones kept tugging me back from the edge of the cliff. Now being home and seeing the signs again, I was reminded this was not just my victory.

The next morning, my wife said, "Okay, dear. It is time for your walk."

I had a wheelchair, a walker, and a cane. I had graduated from the wheelchair. I was in the walker stage even if it was baby steps. A little farther every day. Then I was down to the cane. By October 1, 2020, I was walking fairly well on my own. My wife was happy because soon we could go dancing. We stayed home as I continued to recover, and most events were closed down due to COVID anyway.

In addition to my daily walking, the first task I took up was reviewing the long list of helpers, some who brought food, and others who sent money for the GoFundMe campaign. I wanted to write thank you notes, so I flipped through my address book.

Sometimes, I had to conduct a Google search to find an address. I was not going to let poor vision, shaky hands, or being easily fatigued stop me from the task. These people had sacrificed a piece of their labor to help us out, and nothing short of a personal note would do. I also tried to reach out to some Barnes staff, including doctors with whom I may have shared a bit of attitude. It was not personal. During the dark days, I still had fight in me, and in my confused state, I aimed my irk at the male doctors, particularly Dr. Crippin, Dr. Chapman, and Dr. Korenblat, all of whom I had and have great respect for.

Having cast my bread and positive feelings on the water with my outreach efforts, we planned a Thanksgiving get-together.

The week before Thanksgiving of 2020, we had to cancel the family gathering at a local hotel where the kids could swim, and we could dine. There had been a spike in COVID cases, and it didn't seem to be a prudent plan. Lynne and I shared a quiet dinner at home that day, but I complained about my belly hurting along my incision.

"I don't know what is wrong, honey. I don't feel too bad, but this pain feels like I've been stabbed."

"I'm taking you in to get it looked at. We aren't messing around wondering what is going on, and I talked to Rachel about it already," Lynne said.

"Okay, well, Carle Hospital has a convenient care just down the hall from the ER. So if they needed more tests, they should have everything needed."

Not surprisingly, I was shifted over to the ER, which sent me to, of course, Barnes. *Sheesh.* I thought I was done with this rumbling down I-57, then across I-70 in a hospital wagon.

"Dan, can you come pick me up at Barnes? They have started treating me for shingles, and I'm to be released tomorrow."

"Sure, Doug. I know where the circle drive is from my recent hip surgery, so I will meet you out there."

The next day, I was wheeled out and thought I spied the big Chevrolet 4x4. Then I saw Dan wave. I hoped I could climb up into this beast. With Dan Davis, I would always be traveling in style, but I might need Dan to throw a rope across the seat and help pull me in!

The shingles treatment picked me right up, and we were back to bundling up and going out walking daily. Lynne said, "I see you are able to walk farther and faster. Maybe we can go out soon." She was eager to see if there was any dancing around, but in Illinois, most venues could not have bands or gatherings of any sort because of COVID. Those were the days of carry-out food for bars and restaurants as their only source of revenue. Then, we had a visit from our Danville dance friends, Bill and Diana Jaffe, in the late fall.

We sat on the deck with spacing to be safe per COVID guidelines, and Diana said, "We don't expect any dancing in Danville until spring. We are really excited about getting back to it, though!"

"We will be sure and let you know. And we are so happy that you are improving, Doug," Bill added.

I really couldn't wait to get Lynne out dancing. I might not be able to dance—maybe a slow one—but that didn't matter. She needed and *deserved* some fun after all the chaos she had to endure. I saw a bounce in her step and light in her eyes just hearing our friend's enthusiasm and knowing it wouldn't be long.

The wake of the boat of critical illness impacted my family, and none more so than my wife. In recovery, I was at home *all* the time. No more having the run of the house during the day while I was at work or after I couldn't work anymore, even the frequent visits to dialysis offered her a break. At least I had a man cave in the basement with my TV, laptop, and treadmill.

One day, as she was putting the blood pressure cuff on my arm, I asked about one of my favorite topics, "Honey, tell me a story about life in the Philippines?"

She paused as she recorded my blood pressure readings.

"Well, for any dating, it was required to be chaperoned. I had a young man caller who had come over to visit. While he was there, another suitor came by. An argument ensued as to who should stay, and I wound up telling them both to leave!" The recollection brought a smile and a shake of her head. "My mom gave me a modest scolding about dating two boys!"

Sharing stories and memories helped power us through the long, cold days of winter. The more she talked and reminisced, it seemed to put the scary past further behind us. I brought up an old dating misfire of my own.

"I had a date for homecoming my sophomore year, and the girl had a chance to upgrade her date. She sent me a note with the bad news but also tried for a soft landing as a consolation, as she wrote, 'Doug, don't ever lose that little boy quality.'"

I told Lynne, "She was just trying to make me feel better. Despite some of those sad moments of youth, I had it good growing up. We had a lot of fun boating, fishing, and camping. My main bug-a-boo was my fear of the dark. I would wake in the night, hear the stairs creaking, and be frightened that someone was coming to get me. My imagination ran wild."

"But you said you moved across the street from the cemetery when you moved out to the trailer."

"I was 19 then and didn't think I was afraid of anything. When I found out I was seriously ill, the boyhood fears would come back in the dark, not of who was coming to get me, but I didn't know what was happening in my body and had no control over it. Illness stole the shield of invincibility of youth in a few hours."

We discussed all manner of topics. I'm not implying that we didn't have our conflicts. One day as I was rounding a flight of stairs to the basement, I tripped on a shoe. I caught my fall but instantly cried, "Honey, do you really need so many shoes lined up by the front door?"

"I'll get it taken care of. Don't worry about it." The message was to zip it when it came to her shoes and clothes.

Lynne had plenty of exasperation to go along with living with me. Frequent trips to the doctor, lab, and pharmacy were required to take care of me. Vision problems had me yielding the driving, and I needed a magnifying glass to see anything requiring tight focus. If I tried to thread a fishing line through the eye of a hook? Forget it. Read the small print on labels? "Honey, I need help!" I'm sure she had two hundred other things I did that annoyed her. Most of her frowns came on the dance floor, with me making a misstep or having trouble learning a move. Despite my modest ability in dancing and an endless array of faults, she still accepted me.

In the early spring of 2021, the call came from Janet Mayol. "The Battle Creek Band is playing in the Cross-County Mall in Mattoon on Saturday!" The excitement in her voice was contagious.

"We will try to make it, Janet, thanks." Great, a chance to dance. A chance at some *normalcy.*

We entered the mall to the sounds of the band playing the Statler Brothers' song "Flowers on the Wall." The air smelled of kettle corn, and we made sure to take some home. The crowd was middle age up to seniors, with a few younger couples walking hand in hand and stopping by for a listen.

The band struck an up-tempo tune, and Janet called Lynne

over for a line dance. They were off. I mainly visited with Janet's husband, David, while Janet, Lynne, and Janet's two granddaughters enjoyed line dancing. Janet, as always, was teaching something new. Smiles were abundant among the pandemic-weary gatherers. Wes Wheeler keyed up The Eagles, "Take It To The Limit." I walked to my wife, and we embraced for our first dance. She held me tight as my eyes misted up.

My wife is a nurturer of plants, animals, and kids. She could grow watermelons in the desert. Her efforts at being my "body man" and caretaker were starting to pay off.

The following week, word came too from Bill and Diana that the Dixie Flyers and Captains 3 Bands had dates at the Danville American Legion and the GAO Grotto. Pandemic restrictions were lifting just as I was becoming more able, and we were starting to get our life back.

My Uncle James Cleo Swinford also asked me to visit his church. "Hey, Doug, we prayed for you, and it is a miracle how you have come back. When Erwin and I came to visit you last spring, we had our doubts. I would like you and Lynne to come down and tell your story and have lunch with Betty and me." My Uncle Cleo was nearing his 88th birthday and the last surviving sibling of my dad's. Clean living and strong faith had propelled him to a long life.

"Uncle Cleo, I am excited to come and visit with your church."

I don't know if he told anyone we were coming, so there was a bit of a gasp after my introduction. In church, you often hear those prayer requests of the deathly ill and anticipate that the next news will not be good news. The beautiful First Congregational Church of Marshall, Illinois, was kind enough to host me and let me talk. The sun lit up the stained-glass windows offering a sense of serenity. My reward was the rapt attention the audience allowed me as I shared some of my harrowing tales. Can my rocky path in life lend a hand to someone else by encouragement or inspiration? I hoped to convey something that listeners might relate to. My concluding remarks were simple. "You prayed. I'm here. Praise God!"

In the micro, I was able to make some gestures to express my gratitude. But in the larger sense, I wondered, *what did I owe life?* Time, talent, and treasure had been expended on my behalf. The energy for prayers for me that could have been guided elsewhere. And now I had less ability physically. What could I offer in return? Was there value in doing more to share my experiences? This was on my mind as we continued to adjust to the role of being retired and relating to life in a new way.

As we prepared to celebrate our wedding anniversary in 2021, we discussed the last one on May 29, 2020. I had been under the spell of dreadful mental confusion, furious with the nurses and my wife. The episode allowed one favor: my memory was erased of the brouhaha that ensued when the nurses tried to put on the boxing gloves. My wife recalls, "It took four of us."

I can't imagine many ways to have a worse wedding anniversary. Maybe if my wife saw me running down the street drunk and naked as Will Ferrell's character did in the movie *Old School*. For her, the drunk part would be just as bad as the naked part!

That was but a sad, almost laughable memory now. When our anniversary came around May 29, 2021, we progressed to where we could travel. After all the battles and then steady recuperation, we flew to Florida for a couple of weeks to celebrate. It was our first trip to The Villages retirement community. It did not take long to find the nearby Spanish Springs Square, which had a band every night.

The band Rocky and the Rollers had the crowd engaged, and they started their cover of Wilson Pickett's "Land of a 1000 Dances." It wasn't just the unique lyrics but the spirit that Pickett jolted in the original that the Rollers were now seeking to recreate.

Got to know how to pony
Like Bony Maronie
Mashed potato
Do the alligator…

Na na na na na…

The crowd was singing along now, transformed from the cares of life, the sensations tickling their brains in that area that stores old songs combined with nostalgic feelings to deliver a pleasurable elixir.

I was watching on the sideline, as I still tired easily. Despite sitting, I probably never enjoyed a song more, as I was able to watch the band and follow the lyrics more closely. I watched Lynne dance with a group of gals. A wave of happiness came over me. Yes, the music seduced me, but more so, I was struck by *how damned lucky I was.* The metamorphosis from that babbling tyrant in the hospital to now enjoying life and seeing my wife happy helped me feel renewed in body and spirit.

On to the next song, the chords struck the entry to the song made popular by the Temptations, "My Girl." I could handle this one, slow and soulful, and my wife was looking my way.

The dividends of life continued shortly after the Florida visit as my oldest daughter Ashley and her husband Aaron celebrated the birth of their daughter Aurora in June 2021. Seeing newborn "Rorie," who resembled her mommy, at least to me, produced a unique sense of deja vu. Wasn't Ashley just a baby herself?

After being a patient and needing attention to my needs, 2021 was a time to support others. My mother, in skilled nursing, always enjoyed a visit. So when my big brother Gary was in town from Phoenix for a visit and was going to see Mom in Battle Creek, I was eager to go, too. The visit was more needed to see

Ray Luts, my sister Cheryl's husband, who was fighting kidney cancer and whom I considered my other big brother. Ray was such a part of the family. He and Cheryl had met in the Army and had been part of our family for 50 years. Husband, father of three, and nowadays a grandfather, Ray created stability for my energetic sister to pursue her goals, including resuming her military service in the Air National Guard. Ray, at 6′6″, towered but was a gentle soul. He worked as a payroll manager at Kellogg's. His keen sense of humor was like a lion ready to pounce. When their son Daniel was in college and working during the summers at Kellogg's, he had a debt to pay his dad. Ray had set standards by which he would pay full tuition unless certain grades were not achieved.

Given that Dan had fallen a little short on the grades, Ray quipped, "Do you want to write me a check, or should I set up a payroll deduction for you?" Ray couldn't miss that opportunity. Now, I just wanted to see him. I didn't expect us to discuss "It." I knew Ray wouldn't let on that anything was wrong.

"Honey, I'd like to go to Michigan with Gary and see Ray and visit at Mom's place."

"Go ahead and go. You know, I'm helping with baby Madi right now. Just don't get in trouble with the police like last time!"

"I'm 95 or 96 percent sure we will not engage law enforcement. On second thought, my brother does speed sometimes. But I'm sure we will be fine."

Our last road trip for just the two of us had been almost ten years ago. Gary drove home in his pick-up truck from Phoenix for a visit of friends and family. A fellow Arizonan hearing of his trip to the Midwest contracted him to retrieve a boat from a Michigan seller. My decision to go help pick up the boat was based primarily on the need for us to spend time together, given my brother's serious bout with cancer. We may never have had the chance to do something like this again. So I took a vacation day. I should have known anything with a boat would not be simple from my past experiences with near sinking, actual sinking, and a motor diving into the lake. But we weren't going in a lake, so what could go wrong? No worries this time. All on land.

After a five-hour drive, the 17′ fiberglass watercraft looked in fair shape at first glance. The skiff included an inboard motor and had probably pulled a few skiers in its day. I suppose the pictures on eBay looked decent. I was concerned that the boat was not covered and the interior was mushy and moldy, and the wood frame seats were shot. The boat was junk, and the trailer had severe rust rendering it fragile. The tires were nearly flat, and there was no one home to help us out. Big bro had the paperwork and a bill of sale, so we were legal to take her, and I felt like we were doing someone a favor just to make it disappear. But hey, I watched *American Pickers* and knew some models of cars, boats, and motorcycles had value no matter how old they were and could be refurbished. We checked the tail lights, and of course, they didn't work. The license plate had expired during the time Jimmy Carter was President. We hooked her up and eased to a gas station to air up what was left of the tires.

With tires now inflated, my brother, ever confidant, pulled into a boat shop, and we could see a guy working.

"Yes, I can get to it next week. It is probably just the wiring connection."

Now my brother has powers of persuasion. Maybe it had to do with when he was working construction and moonlighting as a bartender. You learn to connect with people on a different level. I'm sure it was just talking the guy up a little. But the guy came out and fixed the lights. We were on the road, but as it got dark, the lights on the trailer flickered on and off like a Christmas tree.

We made it all the way to Highway 63 near Covington, Indiana, when the cherries lit up.

"Oh shit. I wonder what the gun laws are here? I have my Colt 32 and a bottle of Jack under my seat."

"Oh great, Gary! I can see the inside of a jail coming my way!"

Gary and I had no way of knowing that there had been extensive drug trafficking and money laundering discovered moving up and down Hwy. 63/41. And our blinking lights and expired tag did not set well with the two Indiana State Troopers. They approached one on each side. From the tone, we were clearly suspected of way more than pulling a rotted trailer and pathetic boat down the highway. In my mind, we had nothing to hide, so we could be polite and on our way. Gary didn't feel that way. He felt agitated not just with the stop but with the attitude towards the story he was trying to convey. They asked him to get out of the truck. He's a physically imposing man, broad and powerfully built. They stood clear.

"Do you have any weapons?"

"No." Technically he did not have any weapons *on* him. "Okay, we want you to come back to the car." He was led to the car and questioned.

"How do we know you guys didn't steal that boat? Was anyone there when you took it?"

"I'm just along for the ride. I don't see my brother that often so I just spent the day with him to go get this boat."

"We are bringing our canine unit over here, so if there is anything you want to tell me, now is the time."

"No sir, it's just an old boat somebody saw on eBay and thought was a good deal."

"I need to know if you are getting paid to help with this?" For the first time, the light bulb went off that they thought we were either mules or dupes carrying contraband of some kind.

Thinking this was ludicrous, I went to another level to explain, "Sir, I know you have a job to do. No, I'm not getting paid. If you really want to know, I came today because my brother had cancer a few years ago. Bad. He was in the hospital for nearly a year. I have had my own hard knocks. I had an opportunity to spend a day, a precious day, just with him. Besides that, I can't imagine anyone putting anything of value in that crappy rig."

The German Shepherd quickly bored as he smelled rotten wood, mold, and nothing else. No search of the vehicle was requested.

The Troopers turned friendly, and Gary was now talking fantasy football with his cop. They even called the Illinois State Police to clear us for the rest of our trip. Both well acquainted with the brevity of life, Gary and I had made a memory, just not quite the way we planned!

However, the drive up in 2021 went smoothly, and I enjoyed a great visit with Ray and Mom. It was not that often that Mom got to see all her kids together, but in birth order, Gary, Cheryl, Debbie, and I had assembled.

It was a late summer day as we set up for a picnic by a nearby lake. Our pavilion and tables offered a view of two fishermen and a diver using a spear for carp. Mom beamed in the presence of her kids and son-in-law Ray. The concerns of life were set aside. Oh, I wished we could suspend time in this picture postcard setting. The day capped off a delightful visit for Gary and me.

We said goodbye reluctantly and headed home. We were cruising down I-94 West when a tire blew. As we tried to see if we could put on a spare tire, we hoped law enforcement would come by and maybe cool the traffic off us as the semis blew by. Gary called his daughter Jennifer since it was her car, and she called her roadside service. Over an hour and no help. She called again and said that two elderly men were stranded. Bingo, now we had help from the cops and two tow truck drivers on short order.

Of course, my wife had to tease me, "I didn't think you guys could go anywhere without trouble." I just felt happy that I was able to be there for Ray. He never complained and in fact, was cutting up with paramedics right up to the time we lost him a few weeks after our visit.

After putting Ray to rest in October and navigating the Illinois winter, we returned to the Villages, Florida, in mid-March of 2022. My sister Debbie had recently moved to The Villages and hosted us for our first few days in her new home. Debbie is now retired from the Navy. She is industrious, and if she isn't decorating her house, she is working on making quilts for all new additions to the family. She still makes time for trips up north to see her sons and their families.

"Well, brother, this is the area near the Sawgrass Square that is being built. I will show you guys around, and we can go to Lake Sumpter Square for some dancing tonight!" She was radiant as she spoke of playing Mahjong and attending local festivals. She could walk around the block and make new friends with the other new retirees in her age group.

During our visit, I asked my sister about a poster of my girls she brought to the hospital during my recovery in 1991.

"I had taken that photo of them sitting together on the glider during a visit in March, and after your transplant, I had the poster made for when I visited."

"Well, it captured a moment in time, and everyone who came into my room asked about the kids. If I needed motivation, all I had to do was glance at the poster, which now resides on the wall in our home. At the time, it said to me, 'We need you, Dad.' Now it serves as a reminder of how fast life goes because they have children of the same age!"

After a few days with Sis, we relocated to a hotel within walking distance of the square and recreation center in Spanish Springs. Our friends Dale Eddings and his wife Teresa Clark, formerly living near us in St. Joseph, Illinois, visited from Homosassa, Florida. During the evening, Dale and I discussed his transplant experience of giving a kidney to his sister over 30 years prior. Dale was humble about his having done so.

Dale said, "I was pretty sore, but it didn't take too long to recover."

I told Dale, "I submitted a newspaper article to the local *News-Gazette* in 1991 about my first transplant. I titled it, 'Divine Giving by Mortals.' To me, no one can do what God can, but sharing life through organs is the closest thing humans can do to a divine act. The paper's editor changed the title to 'The Gift that Keeps on Giving.' I was just pleased that he ran it."

After dining, we strolled by the square while a band played

but had to pass on dancing this evening due to the soft but steady rain.

Our friends headed home, and as my wife showered for bed, I looked out the window to watch the raindrops smatter harder on the glass. The palm trees waved gently. No big storms tonight, though. My thoughts turned to my life being extended by someone else's death, which left a lot of questions. This was not a planned donation like with Dale. The unplanned ones came about through dramatic events. Teresa had mentioned earlier about what happened with Ross back home. It offered a glimpse of donation from the other side.

I watched Ross Booker grow up in our church over the last 20 years. His parents did the right things raising him. Ross was on the right track, finishing his college work, and after some local training, he planned to head to the Big Sky country of Montana to work as a diesel mechanic. Yet just a couple of weeks ago, I sat in a high school gym mourning his loss.

High school gyms are a place for cheering at basketball and volleyball and seniors celebrating their graduations with caps flying. But Ross's untimely passing required a large venue. Ross's connections through FFA, St. Joseph Stanton Fire District, and his work with Tatman's towing cast a wide net of friends and coworkers. Ross was finishing a stint with Tatman's when he was cleaning up an accident scene, and an inexperienced driver struck him, causing non-survivable injuries.

By the time I came through the line, his exhausted parents had already greeted for five hours. In a later conversation with his mother, Marita, our church secretary, she said the decision to donate organs was simple, "Ross would do anything to help anyone! It was kind of a way to hold on to what we can of him a little longer. We were able to spend more time with him at the hospital. And he helped many people, one of which received his heart and a kidney. I want to hear his heartbeat again!"

Recalling this conversation had turned the evening somber but uplifting at the same time. Ross's legacy would go on through the good he brought to the world and by his giving spirit. I can see Marita now with the stethoscope and the light in her eyes.

The next morning, Lynne called out, "Honey, you need to get up so we can catch some breakfast and make it to Zumba class this morning."

"Okay, okay, I'll get around." For some reason, I felt just a little bit off. But some coffee, maybe two cups of coffee, a little breakfast, and a light workout would fix it all. I liked the Zumba Gold, as they called the class. I guess that sounded better than Zumba for old people, but it was geared toward our age group. My wife was much better at following the music and motions of the leader. I looked around and tried to follow the strong participants who knew the choreography. I was *that guy* who probably annoyed others since I was out of sync with the class.

After the session at the rec center, we walked back to the hotel.

I told Lynne, "Honey, I'm kind of cold. I know it is 80 degrees, but I feel a chill."

"I'm checking your temperature as soon as we get back to our room." She looked at me and touched her hand on my forehead as we walked.

"What do you see, dear?" She looked at the thermometer.

"It reads 102. What does that mean? Isn't that the same problem as before when you were getting sick?" She started piling blankets on me to keep me from the shaking chills.

I smiled and said with resignation, "I guess we have an unwelcome visitor. I kind of hoped he wouldn't be able to find us."

I wasn't the little boy scared of the dark anymore or frightened of these invisible disease processes. But, at the moment, I was cold, so cold. I found a heat source in my memory bank, and it was lava. Great, powerful waves of lava rolling into the mighty Pacific. I had viewed this collision off the coast of the Big Island of Hawaii while on a cruise. In my mind, the lava gave off heat, not unlike a campfire on a cool night. The stark image of a sky unfettered by city lights, the ocean waves, and the heat of the earth's blood spilling out to be cooled and fractured by the sea made me feel so inconsequential that my fever, now warmed by my image, seemed trivial.

My wife, while concerned, knew the drill all too well. In a few hours, I would usually come out of it. No matter what happened with my condition from here on out, I knew we would experience and deal with it together. I can't explain why knowing she would be there provided so much comfort, but it did.

Whatever pickle in life I have come upon, I have found a way out of it. And when the time comes that all remedies are exhausted, and the earth tires of me walking her, I'll go back to a family reunion in the late 60s at Twin Lakes Park, Paris, Illinois, when my grandfather Adren Swinford, my dad Dale and his brothers Owen, Aaron, James Cleo, and Don took the stage in the pavilion to play guitar and sing the poetic lyrics of Grandpa's favorite hymn, "The Old Rugged Cross."

On a hill far away stood an old rugged cross
The emblem of suffering and shame
And I love that old cross where the dearest and best
For a world of lost sinners was slain

So I'll cherish the old rugged cross (rugged cross)
Till my trophies at last I lay down
I will cling to the old rugged cross
And exchange it some day for a crown

The singing and guitar playing was a little off-key at times during that family reunion, but no more sincere rendition has ever been performed. As young boys, my cousin Marty and I found amusement in their singing and pretended to howl at the moon like wolves. I joked then, but the essence of the message delivered a spiritual, grounding moment in my Christian faith. Their faith anchored mine.

Like the playing and singing, my life has been off-key and missed a note or two. I've heard it said many times, "What a tough guy you are! What a fighter!"

To that, I reply, "Poppycock." I don't entertain pain any better than anyone else. Pain and suffering have been a toll I have had to pay for the rewards of the happy parts of life. Besides, in a sense, I have already won this grappling match with my adversary. Try to take me away from raising my young daughters? Failed. Keep me from my charge to get my baby Rachel through high school? Get out of my way! Barring me from enjoying the treat of grandkids and leisure with my wife? Not so fast. Every hour and every day has been hard fought for and is a triumph.

When I see my wife smiling on the dance floor, hear my grandkid's joy for life, or hear them call me Grandpa Doug, Pa Pa Doug, Ta-Ta, or Pop Pop, it *moves* me. It's all I need.

It's June 22, 2022, and 31 years removed from my first transplant. I step out the door for an early morning walk to beat the summer heat. I smell the blossoms on the tree right outside our front door. My wife's flower beds offer a pleasant aroma as well. I walk past the natural peace of a nearby cornfield. I reflect on my life being doubled in length by dramatic measures. Being there for my family and treating my fellow man well is all I can do in return. I have had a few dents in life, some never completely repairable. But if I'm ever tempted to melancholy over it, I recall the words my date-breaking girl in high school said, "Doug, don't ever lose that little boy quality."

And I haven't.

THE END

MEMORIES

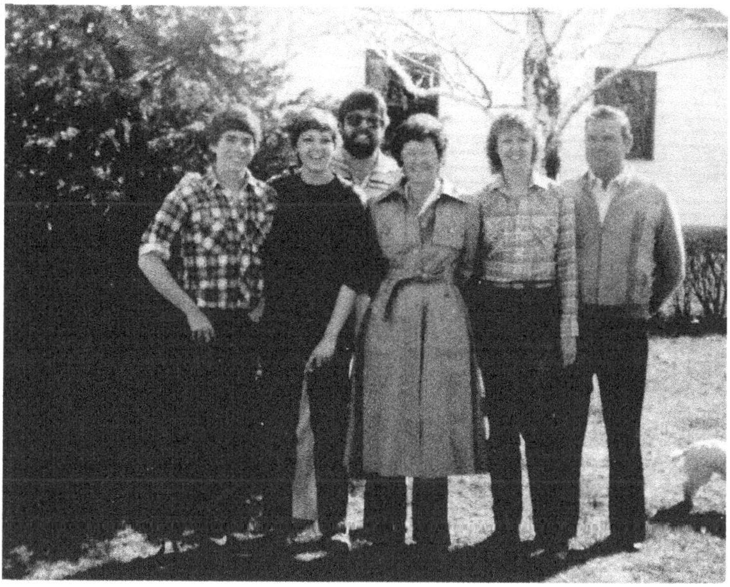

Family Picture, 1977

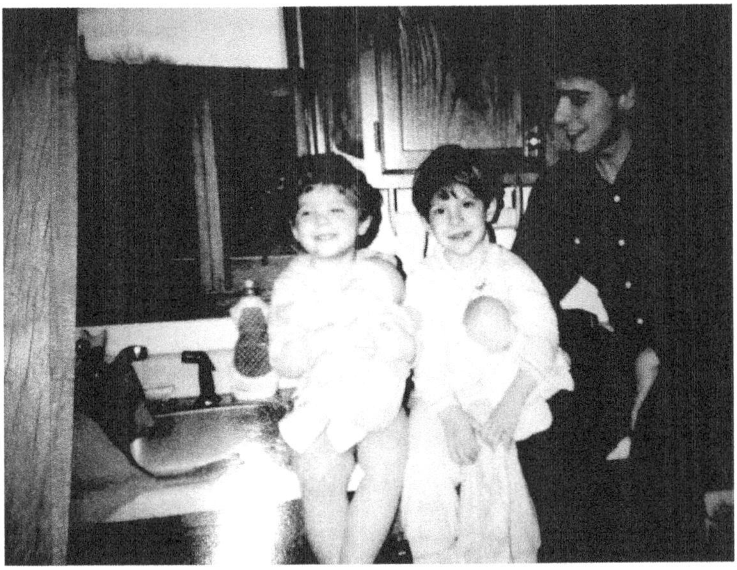

Jessi, Ashley, and me before Rachel came

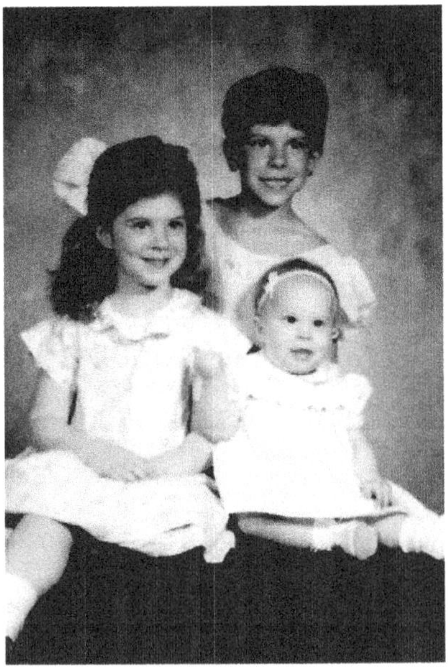

A new addition to the family

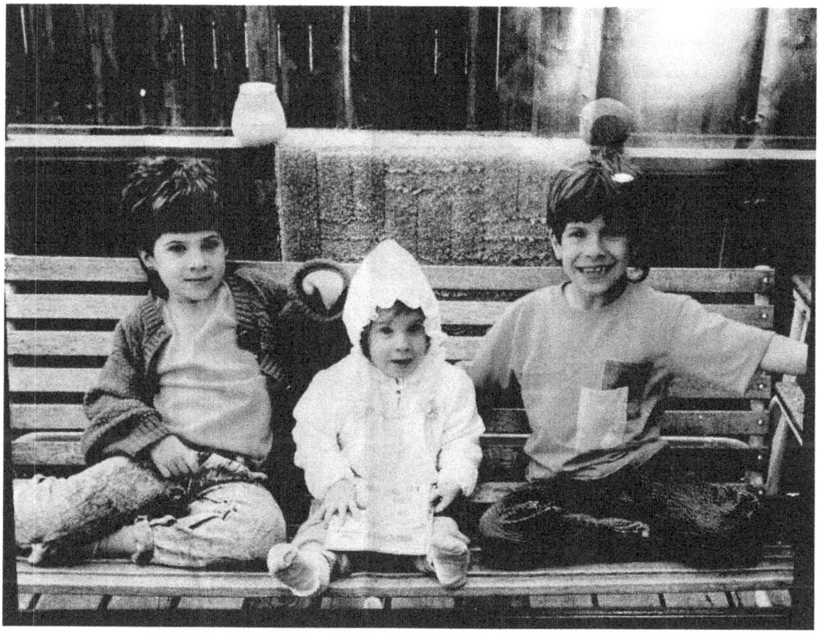

Hospital wall poster

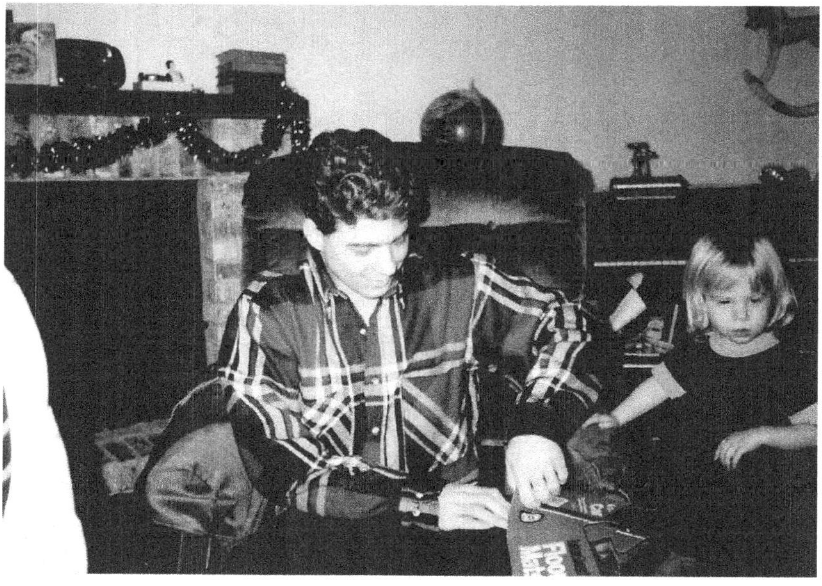

Christmas, 1991

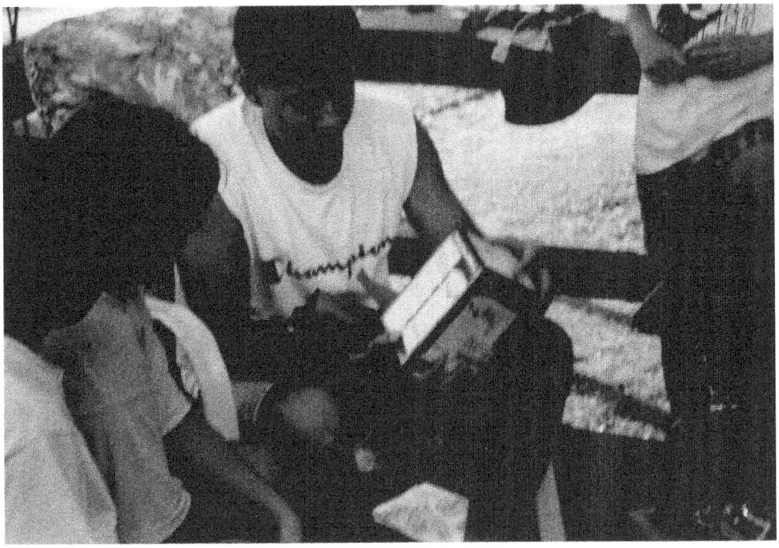

Father's Day at my parent's Arkansas home, 1994

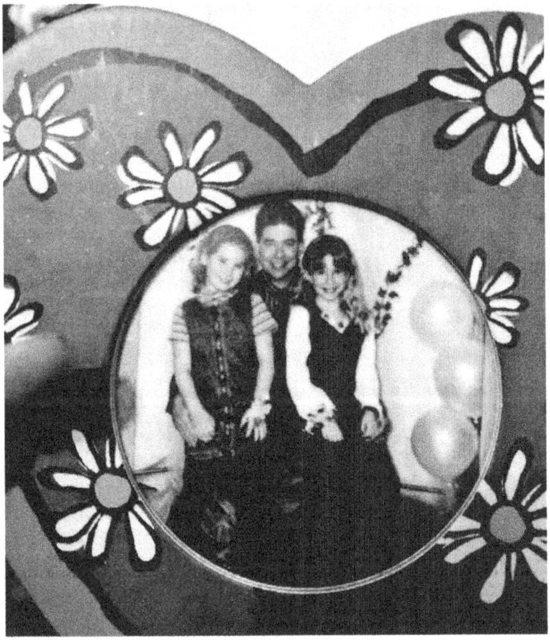

Daddy-daughter dance with Rachel and her friend Christina

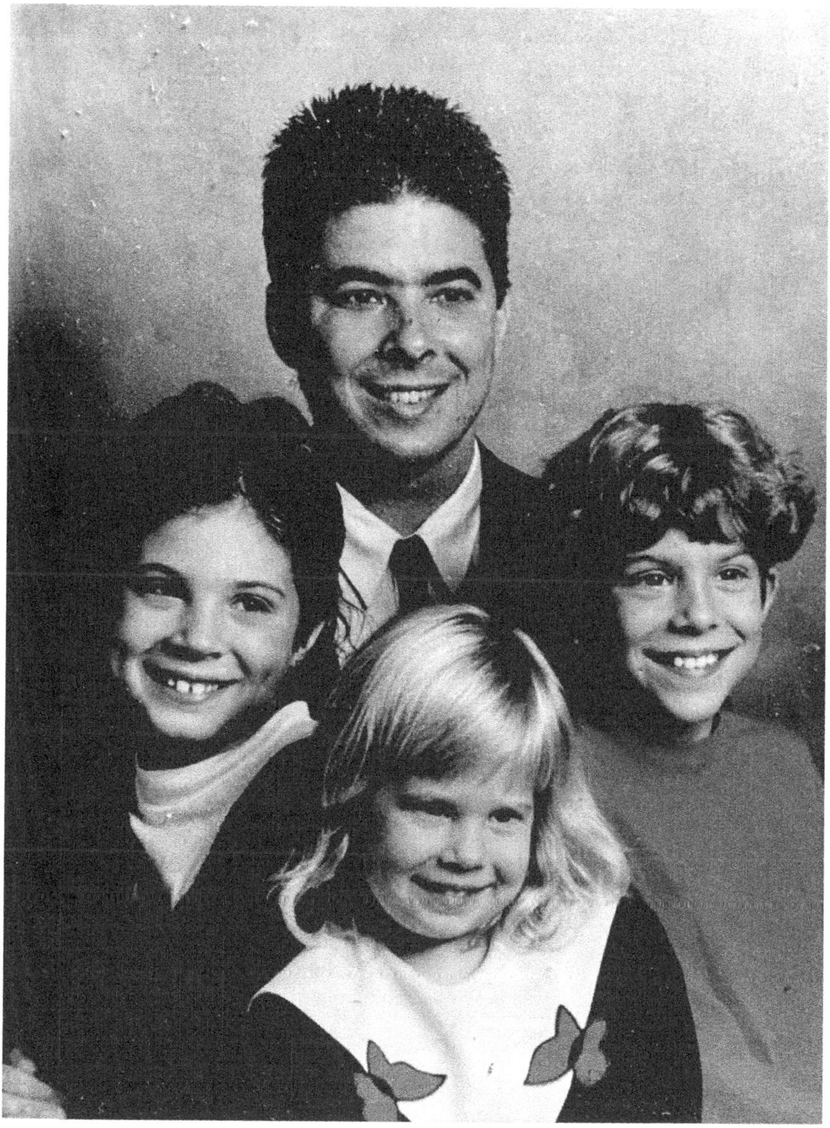

A father and his daughters

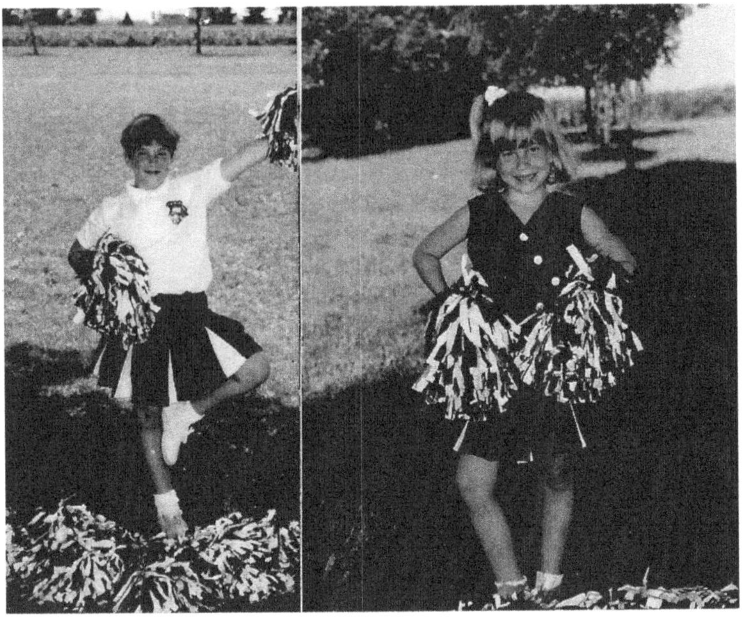

Youth Football Cheerleaders, 1996

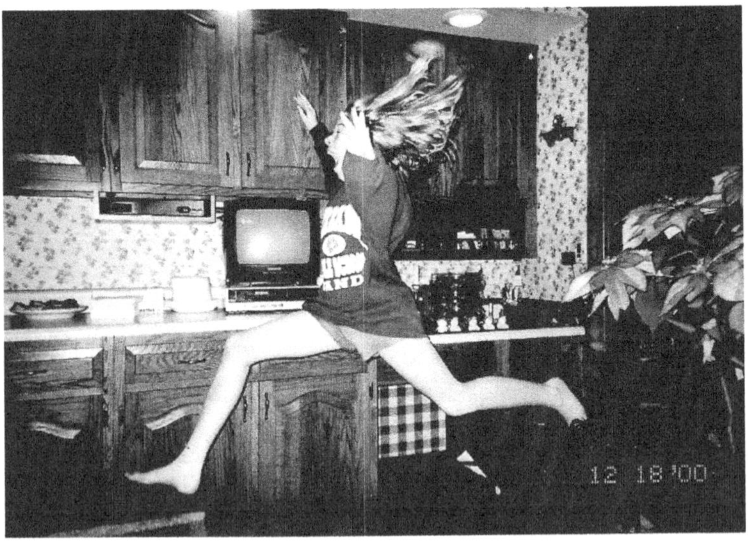

Rachel leaping… general mayhem in our household!

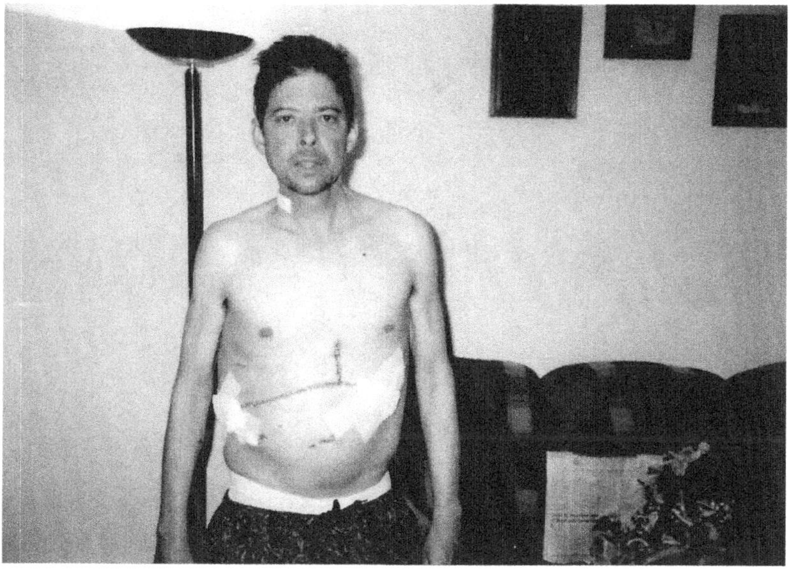

Transplant aftermath, 2004

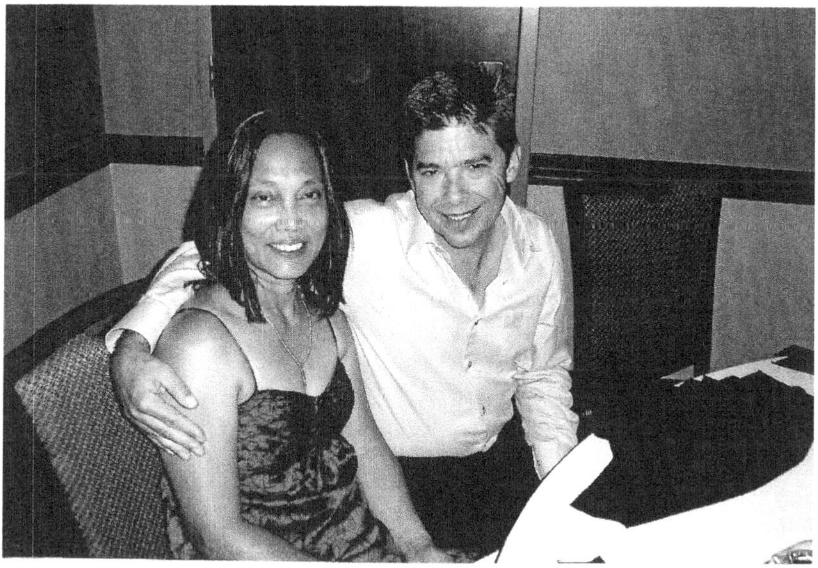

A new couple, 2009

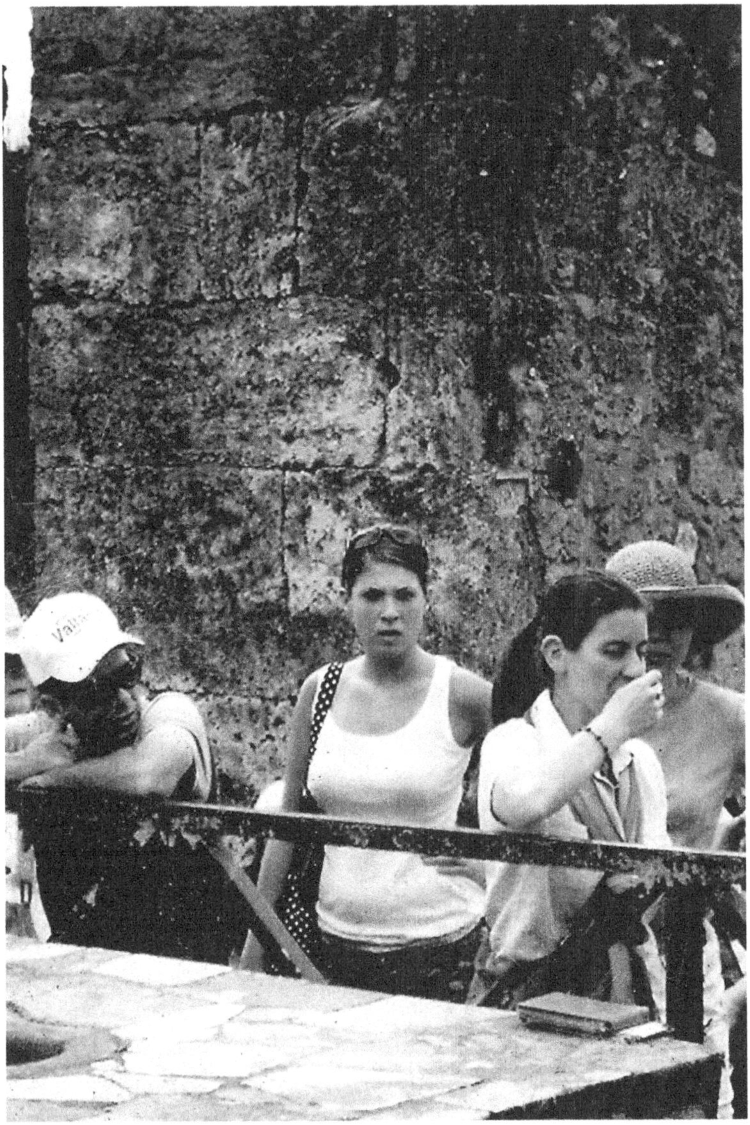

Jessi and me during a hot day in Pompeii

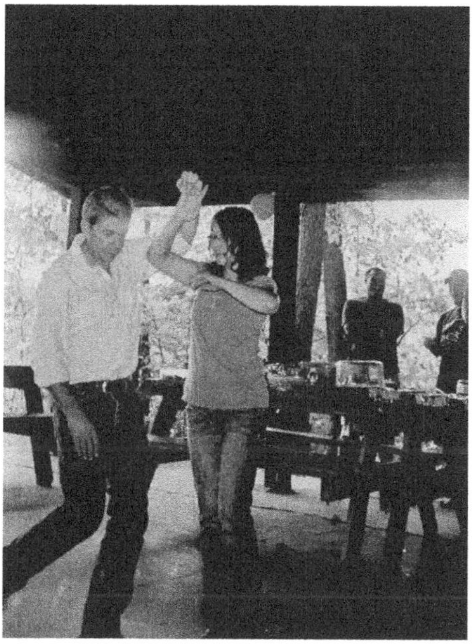

Fil-Am picnic dance

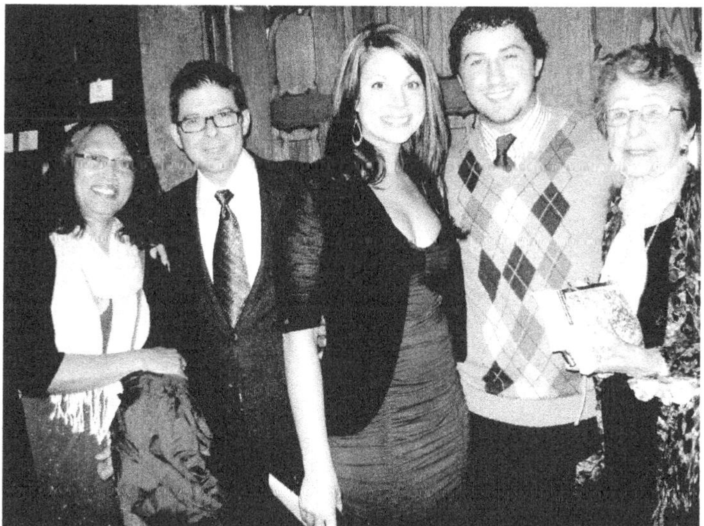

Lynne, me, Jessi, Tony, and Mom

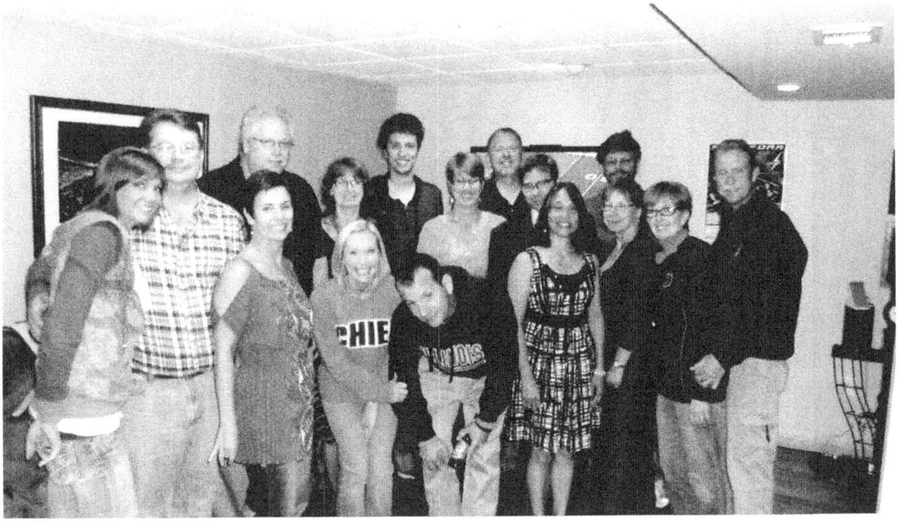

Storm cellar, New Year's Eve

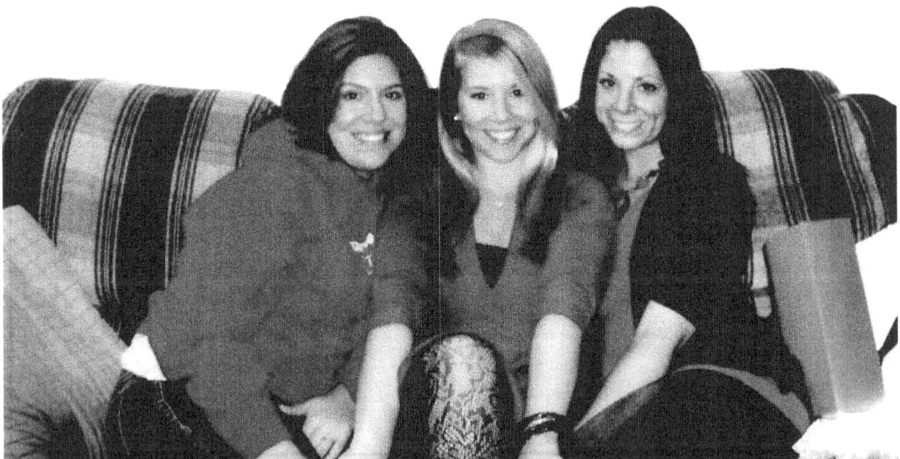

Ashley, Rachel, Jessi

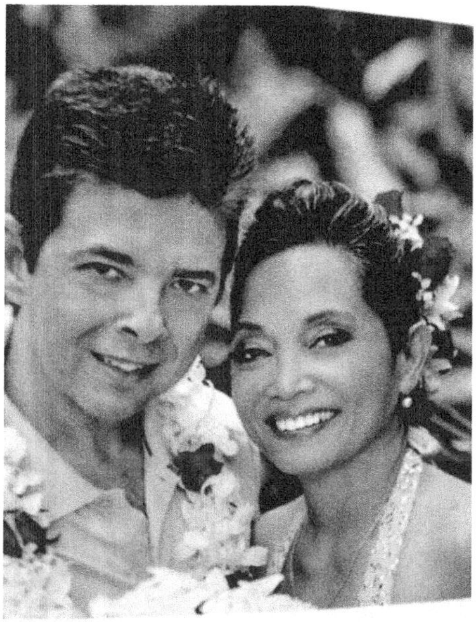

Wedding day, Hawaii 2013

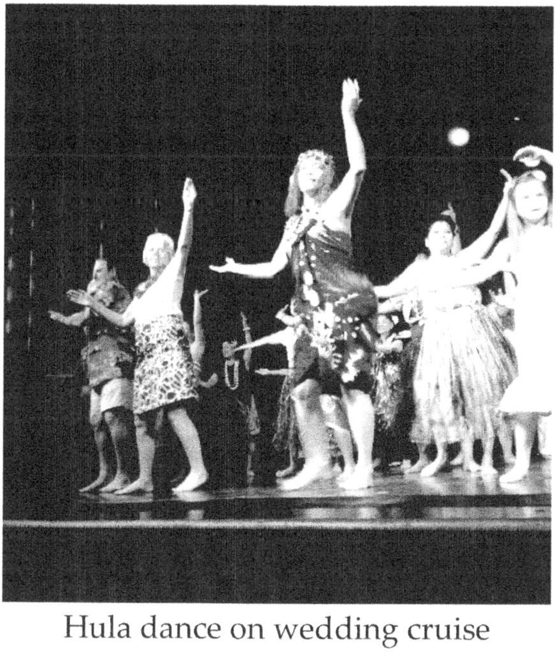

Hula dance on wedding cruise

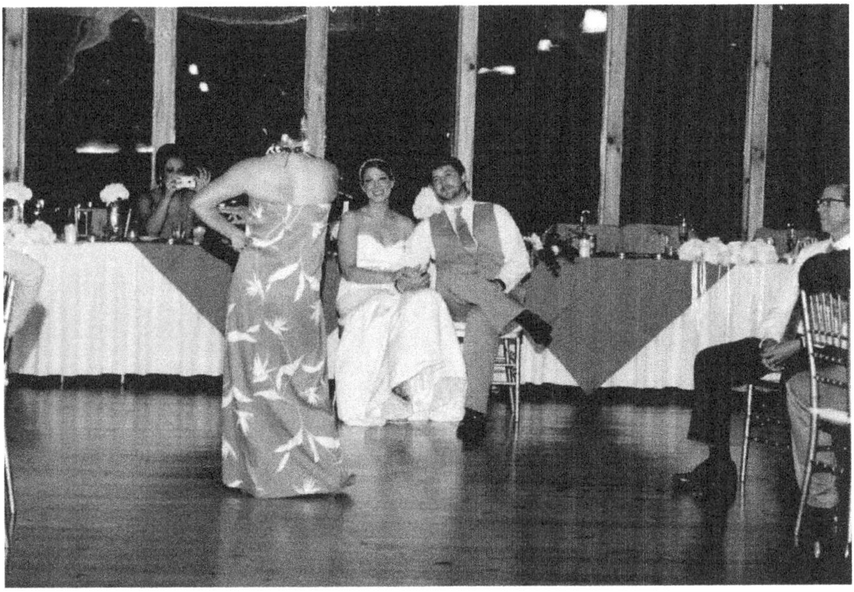

Jessi and Tony wedding, 2015

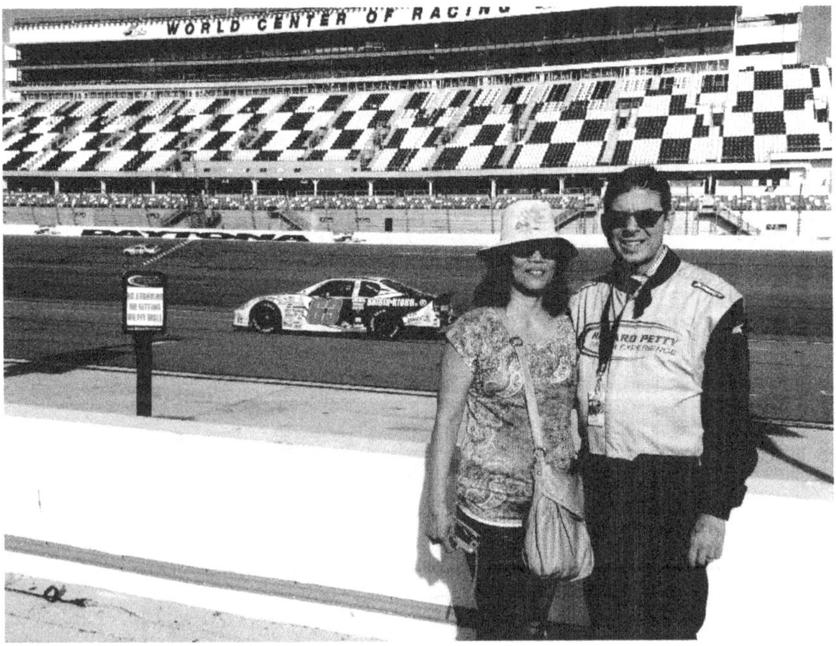

Daytona Speedway, bucket list item!

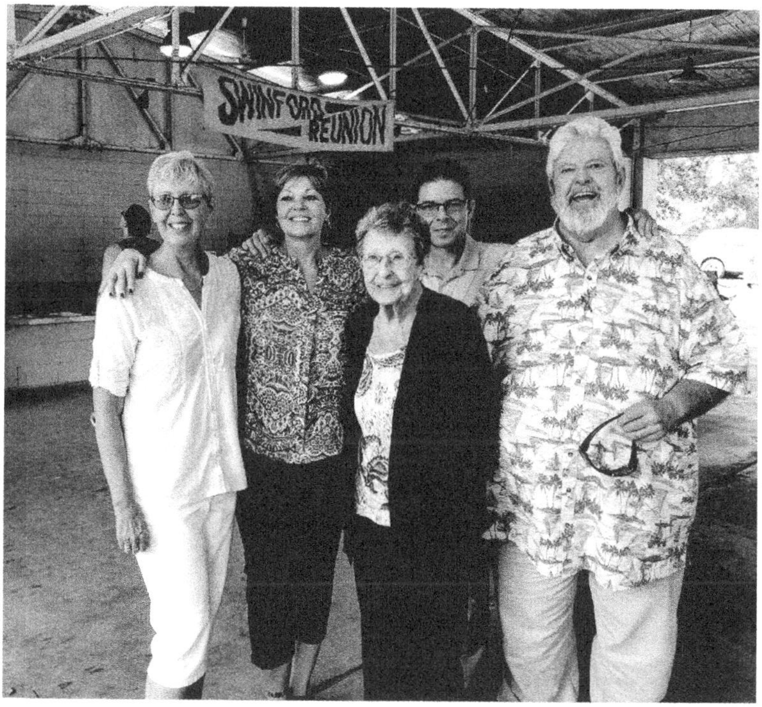

Mom and siblings

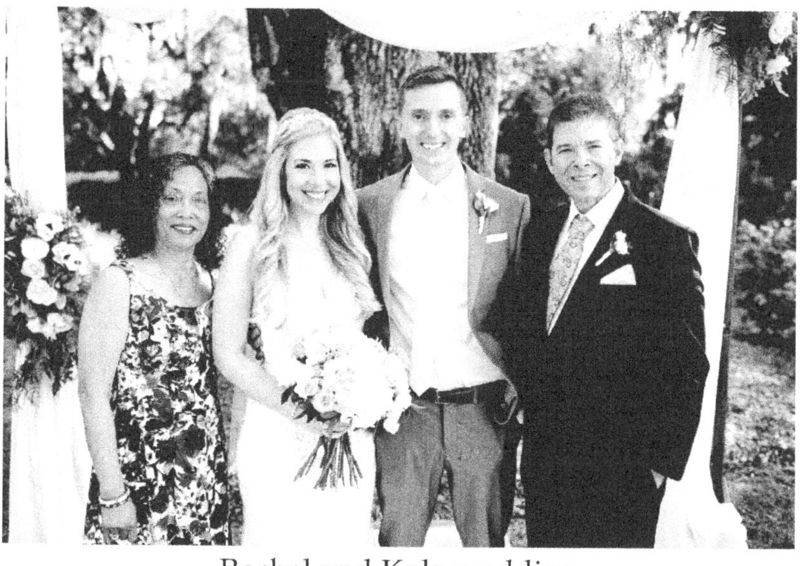

Rachel and Kyle wedding

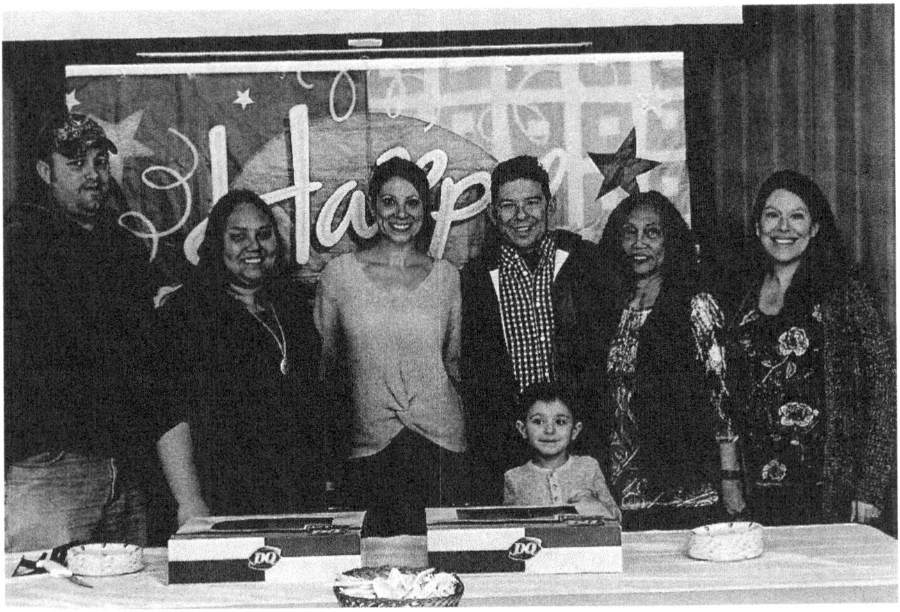

Retirement Party, 2019

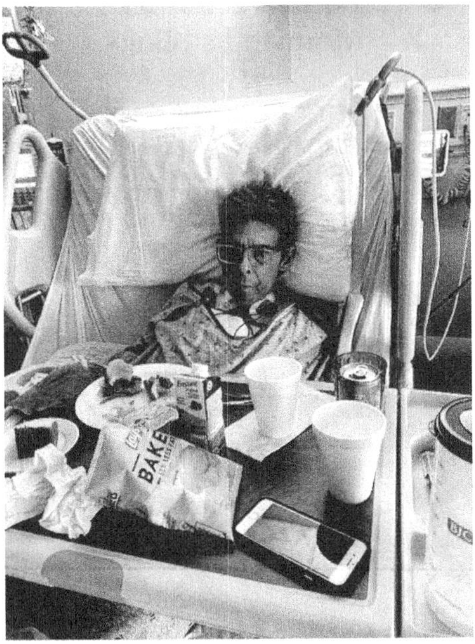

Hanging on, June 2020

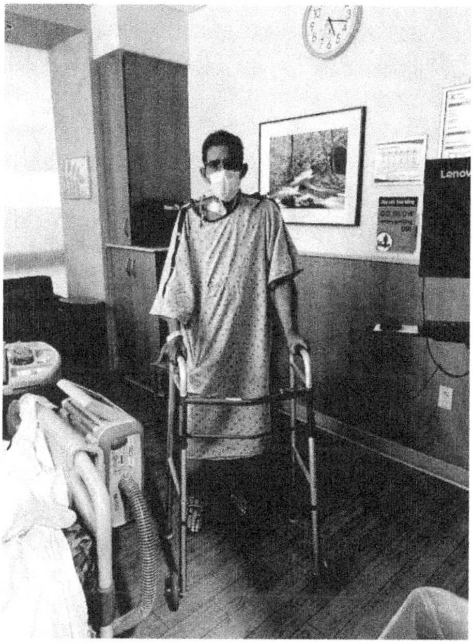

New wheels, August 2020

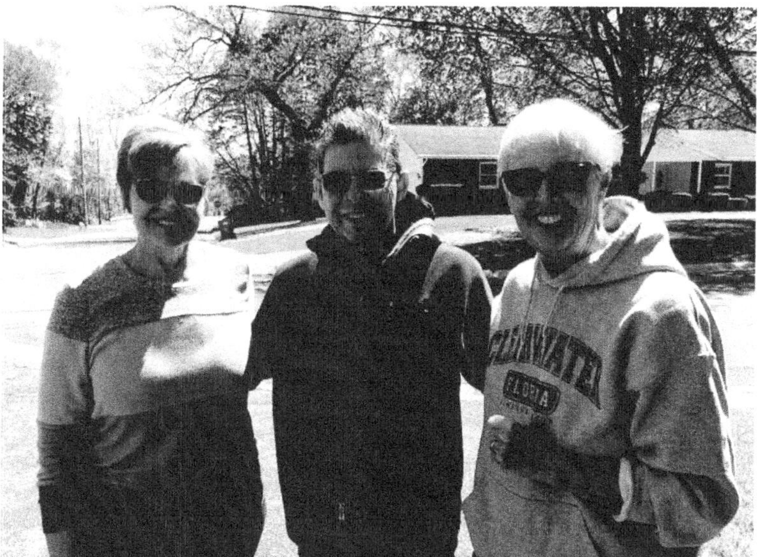

My sisters, Battle Creek, Michigan, 2021

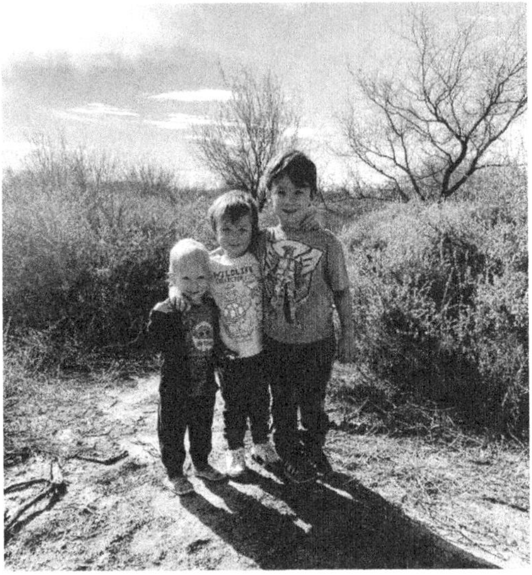

Everett, Giio, and Vinny, El Paso, Texas, December 2021

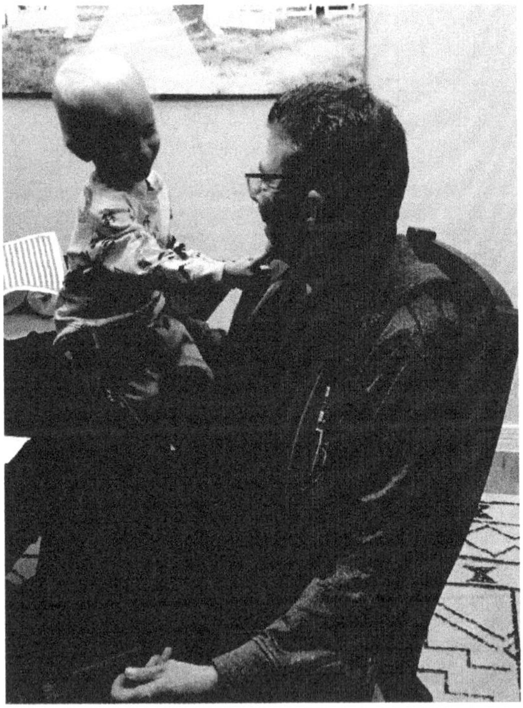

Everett and Pop Pop, Christmas 2021

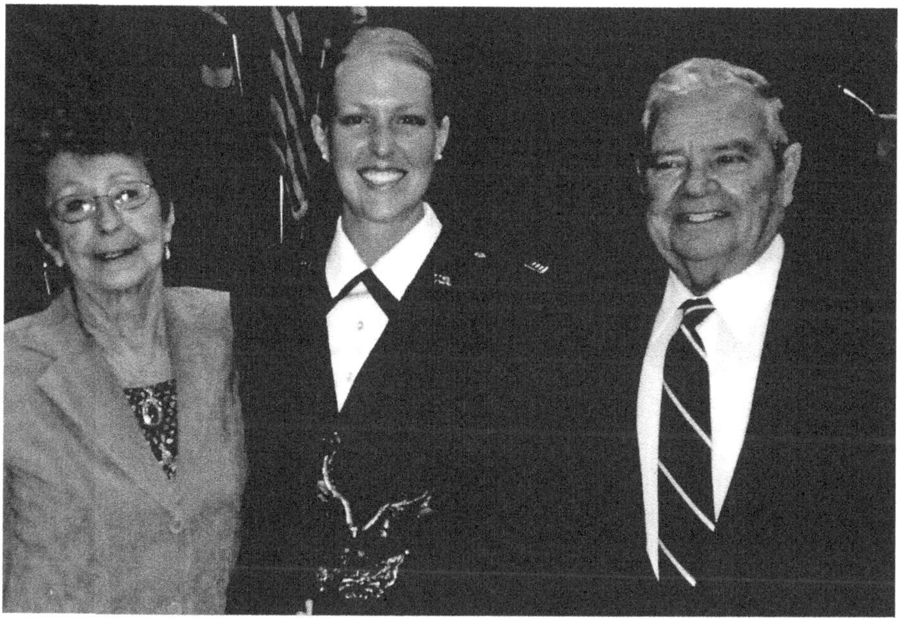

Mom, Lindsey Luts, and Dad

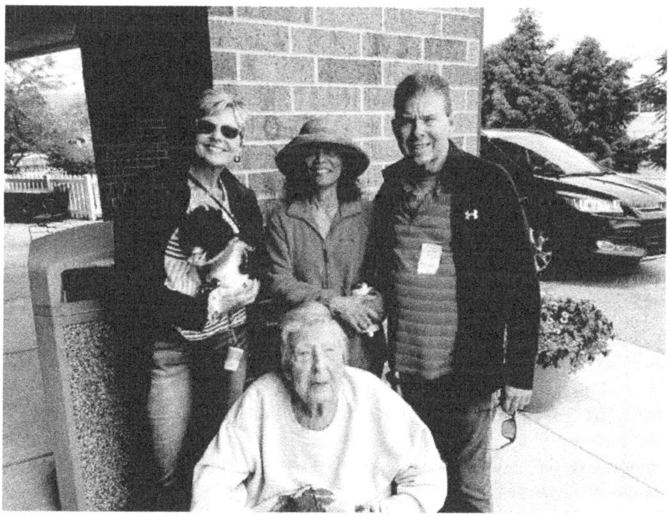

Mom, sister, Debbie, Lynne, and me

ACKNOWLEDGMENTS

Writing your first book is a little like if you tried to build your own house; most of us would run into a lot of struggles and need professional contractors to step in. And that's what I did.

Margo L. Dill from Editor-911 Writer Services helped me get started with the basics needed to organize the book and provided developmental editing. I appreciate her patience in sifting through my initial efforts. Margo recommended I find someone to help me further the project and help with the publishing process.

Robert Henry from Right Hand Publishing provided further editing, proofreading, page design, and assistance with the entire publishing process. Robert coached me through the endless details required to make it all happen. He also referred me to Robin Locke Monda (Locke Monda Graphic Arts) to create a professional book cover, and she gave me six wonderful options, making it difficult to pick!

Fred Olds, a long-time friend and author of children's books, read my rough draft and encouraged me to make a go of it and connected me with Margo. Fred has been a cheerleader all along.

Another author, my late Uncle Don Swinford inspired me with his writing numerous books including one about my dad titled *D.A.L.E.* His wonderful books and steadfast dedication to the craft continues to inspire me!

There are so many people I would like to mention that are not captured in any scenes of the book. Invariably and unintentionally, I would leave people out. But I would be remiss not to mention the guys and gals from my Illinois Power and Ameren tenure from 1979-2019 from both the Champaign and Danville operating centers. The heat, the cold, the mud, the storms, and the emergencies impacted both field and office personnel to give us a common bond. Many of those relationships remain strong.

My wife Lynne encouraged me from the start and allowed me the time to work on the project without complaint.

My siblings all provided support. Debbie and Gary provided commentary and Cheryl became my primary "reader." I was very fortunate to gain her insight as she had the knowledge of the situation that my other editors didn't have. For example, she might say, "Brother, I remember you were way more upset about that situation than the way you wrote it!" With her help, I could dig deeper into my memory and make changes that better represent the truth.

And then I have my "listeners," who listened patiently as I rattled on and on about the project, asked for their opinion on titles, or asked them to look at the book cover options. Of course, my daughters, their husbands, and in-laws offered productive and consistent feedback. Our dance friends were good sports as well. Nancy Brain and Tom Passo were supportive and offered positive feedback.

When I shared with Lee and Jan Gurga, I found that Lee had authored a book about Japanese poetry. Lee and Jan also provided a final proofread, for which I'm very grateful. Other dance friends chimed in with Bill and Jan Keeler shared about a crime thriller that Bill had authored and self-published. When I explained my book to Wes and Marj Seitz, Wes chuckled, recalling an economics textbook he had written, and commented that he made about a penny an hour on the project. Wes also helped expand our dancing skills and make new friends by inviting us to the University Club. I had known Barb and Warren Johnson from dancing and cruises, and Barb was very supportive and just a phone call away if I needed her. Former co-worker Alan Ellis patiently listened over breakfast meetings; he plans to write his own book with the help of his friend Sue. Sue will probably deserve the author credit on that book. I tried not to wear anyone out with endless details. Still, I prevailed upon my captive audiences, which also included my Sunday school class as well as the "Breakfast with the old people" retirement group.

And my Facebook helpers! I put out four title suggestions as well as asked for ideas. An avalanche of good ideas came forth.

Four suggestions provided ideas for chapter titles: "Dying to Live," "Running from the Darkness," "Don't Forget to Dance," and "The Rock Keeps Rolling" were spurred by ideas by Linda Oldham, Connie Lewis Knight, Sandi Bennett Schopp, and Tracy Bailey respectively. From the lighter side, my nephew Jeff Luts offered the following: "Doug Life," "Bone Doug in Harmony," "Dig Doug," and "Prescription Pharmaceutical Doug."

And to all the people who took an interest and read the book, I feel so privileged to be able to share a part of my life with you. I hope it left you with positive feelings, which was my goal. While it's been a unique challenge, it has been a rewarding experience to bring this to you!

Any comments or questions can be sent to my e-mail at
dmichael13@comcast.net

Made in the USA
Monee, IL
03 August 2023

40429206R00142